DERMATOLOGY – LABORATORY AND CLINICAL RESEARCH

ATOPIC DERMATITIS

FROM DIAGNOSIS TO TREATMENT

DERMATOLOGY – LABORATORY AND CLINICAL RESEARCH

Additional books and e-books in this series can be found on Nova's website under the Series tab.

DERMATOLOGY – LABORATORY AND CLINICAL RESEARCH

ATOPIC DERMATITIS

FROM DIAGNOSIS TO TREATMENT

ANDREAS MAUR
EDITOR

nova
Medicine & Health
New York

Library of Congress Cataloging-in-Publication Data

Names: Maur, Andreas, editor.
Title: Atopic dermatitis : from diagnosis to treatment / Andreas Maur, editor.
Description: New York : Nova Science Publishers, [2020] | Series: Dermatology - laboratory and clinical research | Includes bibliographical references and index. |
Identifiers: LCCN 2020039689 (print) | LCCN 2020039690 (ebook) | ISBN 9781536185201 (hardcover) | ISBN 9781536186413 (adobe pdf)
Subjects: LCSH: Atopic dermatitis.
Classification: LCC RL243 .A864 2020 (print) | LCC RL243 (ebook) | DDC 616.5/1--dc23
LC record available at https://lccn.loc.gov/2020039689
LC ebook record available at https://lccn.loc.gov/2020039690

Published by Nova Science Publishers, Inc. † New York

CONTENTS

PREFACE

Atopic dermatitis is a chronic inflammatory skin disease that is characterized by xerosis, eczema lesions with skin barrier defects, and severe itch. This compilation describes recent advances in our understanding of intractable itch mechanisms and the development of antipruritic therapies in in this condition. Additionally, the authors summarize the current developments in understanding the comorbidities of atopic dermatitis.

Insight into various emerging therapies along with currently approved treatments is provided. Some proposed interventions are presented regarding the population group that can benefit the most according to the severity of the symptoms, the mechanism of action of the intervention and the possible adverse effects.

The authors use Pentaherbs Formula to educate to readers on efforts in Traditional Chinese Medicine research to adopt this historic and unique complementary medicine as a safer and scientific-based therapy for atopic dermatitis.

In closing, *Atopic Dermatitis: From Diagnosis to Treatment* focuses on topical corticosteroids that are commonly used by dermatologists and general physicians to treat selected difficult dermatoses effectively.

Chapter 1 - Atopic dermatitis (AD) is a chronic inflammatory skin disease that is characterized by xerosis, eczema lesions with skin barrier defects, and severe itch. Intractable itch with AD is generally resistant to conventional therapy, such as H_1-antihistamines. Patients with AD also develop itch hypersensitivity, which results in an itch-scratch cycle. Intractable itch causes sleep disturbances and psychological stress (depression, anxiety, and even suicidal feelings) in AD patients, which have a negative impact on performance in school or at work and reduce quality of life (QOL). Reduced QOL further diminishes motivation to pursue an industrious life and social activities, thereby affecting socioeconomic activity. The underlying neuro-immunological mechanisms of itch have been attracting increasing attention and have become a vibrant and rapidly advancing field of research. Recent studies reported that cytokine receptors expressed by sensory nerve fibers were predominantly associated with itch sensitization. Furthermore, barrier defects have been shown to activate Th2 immune pathways and promote the production of Th2 cytokines (such as interleukin [IL]-4, IL-5, IL-13, and IL-31) in skin. Clinically, biological therapies, such as dupilumab (anti-IL-4 receptor a monoclonal antibody), were found to attenuate pruritus as well as skin inflammation in AD patients. Clinical trials on nemolizumab (anti-IL-31 receptor A monoclonal antibody) and Janus kinase (JAK) inhibitors (e.g., delgocitinib, ruxolitinib, and tofacitinib) demonstrated that the amelioration of pruritus in AD patients. In January 2020, topical delgocitinib, which inhibits all members of the JAK family (JAK1-3 and tyrosine kinase 2), was approved for the treatment of AD in Japan. Intraepidermal nerve fibers or spinal glial cells contribute to itch hypersensitivity in a disease state-dependent manner. New antipruritic approaches against AD are targeting immune and neural molecules or cells. This chapter describes recent advances in our understanding of intractable itch mechanisms and the development of antipruritic therapies in AD.

Chapter 2 - Atopic dermatitis is a common chronic inflammatory skin disorder that affects children and adults worldwide. Given the frequent association with elevated serum levels of immunoglobulin E, atopic dermatitis usually encompasses a personal or family history of atopy, which represents a group of disorders including allergic rhinitis, asthma, food allergy and eosinophilic esophagitis. In addition to the well-established knowledge of the relationship between atopic dermatitis and other atopic disorders, increasing evidence has shown that patients with atopic dermatitis also appear to be at higher risk for numerous nonallergic comorbidities, such as infections, neuropsychiatric conditions, metabolic syndrome, cardiovascular diseases, autoimmune diseases and malignancy. Although the pathologic mechanisms behind their links are still largely controversial, these findings suggest cutaneous and systemic immune dysregulation in atopic dermatitis and highlight the possibility that this disease may be more of a systemic disorder than previously perceived. Managing clinicians should be aware of these potential associations and incorporate them into holistic approaches in treating patients with atopic dermatitis. This chapter summarizes the current insight and development in understanding the comorbidities of atopic dermatitis.

Chapter 3 - Atopic dermatitis (AD) is a chronic and pruritic skin condition which affects 10 – 20% of the population worldwide. It can be characterized by pruritus, erythema, vesiculation, exudation, excoriation, crusting, scaling and sometimes lichenification. AD usually starts during infancy or early childhood, and is the commonest childhood skin disease. The lifetime prevalence of AD is estimated to 15-30% in children, and 2-10% in adults. In the past 3 decades, the incidence of AD has increased by 2- to 3-fold in industrialized countries, and this prevalence continues to increase. As its causes are still poorly understood, the management of AD always presents a great challenge to all clinicians. Although etiology of AD is unclear, genetic factors play a significant role in contributing its prevalence. Nevertheless, recent increase in AD prevalence suggests complex interaction between environmental factors and susceptibility genes may also result in clinical expression of the disorder. Current therapeutic approaches of AD often focus on symptomatic relief rather than cure, and the long-term treatment objectives for AD are aimed at reducing the clinical manifestations, minimizing relapses, and modifying the disease course. These approaches comprise basic skin care for cutaneous rehydration with liberal use of emollients, intermittent use of anti-inflammatory therapy for acute flares and avoidance of triggering factors. Recent increases in the use of TCM, especially in Asia may provide an alternative treatment option. However, the beneficial effects of TCM on AD have not been consistently demonstrated. This book chapter aims to provide a review of AD, from its diagnosis to its recent advances in the treatment options.

Chapter 4 - Atopic dermatitis (AD) is a common chronic, pruritic, inflammatory dermatosis that affects the population worldwide. AD is primarily characterized by skin barrier dysfunction and is mediated by a cutaneous immune response. To date, the primary therapy for AD inflammation is still the use of topical corticosteroids, while severe refractory and inadequately controlled AD cases are treated with systemic immune-suppressive medications. Growing knowledge of the pathogenesis of AD has allowed recent development of more targeted topical and systemic therapies by supplementing barrier function, suppressing inflammation or inhibiting elevated T helper (Th) 2 cytokines (interleukin (IL)-4, IL-5, IL-13, IL-33, thymic stromal lymphopoietin and their receptors) or Th22/Th17 cytokines. In addition, there are also other emerging therapies, such as inhibitors of phosphodiesterase, Janus kinase, immunoglobulin E and histamine, and antipruritic agents. Besides, because dysbiosis in the skin microbiome enables *Staphylococcus aureus* colonization, which exacerbates inflammation in AD, the transplantation of commensal strains and anti-staphylococcal treatment targeting *Staphylococcus aureus* are also promising therapies under investigation. This chapter provides insight into various emerging therapies along with currently approved treatments for AD.

Chapter 5 - Multiple treatments have been proposed for atopic dermatitis, however not all of them are useful for all people. In this chapter, the authors review some proposed interventions in the management of atopic dermatitis and the population group that can benefit the most according to the severity of the symptoms, the mechanism of action of the intervention and the possible adverse effects. Dogs share many common characteristics with humans in the pathogenesis of the disease, perhaps due to their mutual coexistence. At the final of the chapter the authors present a comparison of the therapies used in humans and their usefulness (or not) in pets as part of integrative medicine.

Chapter 6 - Being considered as the first step in the "atopic march," atopic dermatitis (AD) may progressively develop from a typical sequence of AD, food allergy, allergic rhinitis and asthma. Patients with AD may need to go through great lengths in order to achieve some relief, while others may even be at the expense of their long-term health. Continuous efforts have been, and are still being made in the search for alternative or adjunct therapies for relieve or treatment. Traditional Chinese Medicine (TCM) has a long history for use in allergies and AD. TCM utilizes herbs that are combined in a prescription in accordance to Chinese medicine theories. With the increasing demand for TCM in recent decades, its efficacy and safety have been frequently questioned. Pentaherbs Formula (PHF) is a Chinese herbal oral concoction modified from an ancient TCM formulation. Previous clinical trials demonstrated its potential in children with moderate-to-severe AD. *In vitro* and *in vivo* experiments further confirmed its efficacy and provided insight on the underlying mechanisms which contribute to the observed beneficial effects. The promises of PHF on AD both clinically and pre-clinically have led to the further exploration of its potential as topical therapy from simple topical lotions, to encapsulation with hydrogel conjugation or even application onto the natural fabric as textile-based transdermal therapy. This chapter will utilize PHF as an example, to illustrate to readers on efforts and stages taken in TCM research in an attempt to adopt this historic and yet unique complementary medicine to become a safer and scientific-based therapy for wider applications.

Chapter 7 - Atopic dermatitis (AD) also known as atopic eczema or eczema. It is a chronic inflammatory, pruritic skin disease that significantly affected the quality of life (QOL) for both patients and families. Topical corticosteroids (TCS) are commonly used by dermatologists and general physicians to treat selected difficult dermatoses effectively. The available range of formulations and potency gives flexibility to treat all groups of patients, different phases of disease, and different anatomic sites. However, majority people are afraid when come to TCS treatments. This fear is due to side effects of improper use of TCS by dermatologists, general physicians, and patients. To maximise therapeutic benefit and minimize the adverse effect, it is necessary to consider the choice of TCS during the diagnosis as well as steroid potency, delivery vehicle, frequency of administration, duration of treatment, and side effects. Benefits of rational and ethical use, danger of overuse and misuse for non-medical, especially for cosmetic purposes, should be clearly evaluate before prescription.

In: Atopic Dermatitis
Editor: Andreas Maur
ISBN: 978-1-53618-520-1

Chapter 1

RELIEF FROM INTRACTABLE ITCH IN ATOPIC DERMATITIS

Yayoi Kamata[1,2], Mitsutoshi Tominaga[1,2] and Kenji Takamori[1,2,3,*]

[1]Juntendo Itch Research Center (JIRC), Institute for Environmental and Gender-Specific Medicine, Juntendo University Graduate School of Medicine, Urayasu, Chiba, Japan

[2]Anti-Aging Skin Research Laboratory, Juntendo University Graduate School of Medicine, Urayasu, Chiba, Japan

[3]Department of Dermatology, Juntendo University Urayasu Hospital, Urayasu, Chiba, Japan

---

* Corresponding Author's E-mail: ktakamor@juntendo.ac.jp.

Abstract

Atopic dermatitis (AD) is a chronic inflammatory skin disease that is characterized by xerosis, eczema lesions with skin barrier defects, and severe itch. Intractable itch with AD is generally resistant to conventional therapy, such as H_1-antihistamines. Patients with AD also develop itch hypersensitivity, which results in an itch-scratch cycle. Intractable itch causes sleep disturbances and psychological stress (depression, anxiety, and even suicidal feelings) in AD patients, which have a negative impact on performance in school or at work and reduce quality of life (QOL). Reduced QOL further diminishes motivation to pursue an industrious life and social activities, thereby affecting socioeconomic activity. The underlying neuro-immunological mechanisms of itch have been attracting increasing attention and have become a vibrant and rapidly advancing field of research. Recent studies reported that cytokine receptors expressed by sensory nerve fibers were predominantly associated with itch sensitization. Furthermore, barrier defects have been shown to activate Th2 immune pathways and promote the production of Th2 cytokines (such as interleukin [IL]-4, IL-5, IL-13, and IL-31) in skin. Clinically, biological therapies, such as dupilumab (anti-IL-4 receptor α monoclonal antibody), were found to attenuate pruritus as well as skin inflammation in AD patients. Clinical trials on nemolizumab (anti-IL-31 receptor A monoclonal antibody) and Janus kinase (JAK) inhibitors (e.g., delgocitinib, ruxolitinib, and tofacitinib) demonstrated that the amelioration of pruritus in AD patients. In January 2020, topical delgocitinib, which inhibits all members of the JAK family (JAK1-3 and tyrosine kinase 2), was approved for the treatment of AD in Japan. Intraepidermal nerve fibers or spinal glial cells contribute to itch hypersensitivity in a disease state-dependent manner. New antipruritic approaches against AD are targeting immune and neural molecules or cells. This chapter describes recent advances in our understanding of intractable itch mechanisms and the development of antipruritic therapies in AD.

Keywords: intractable itch, skin barrier, neuroimmune mechanism, antipruritic therapy

1. Introduction

Atopic dermatitis (AD) is a chronic skin disease characterized by eczematous skin lesions, epidermal barrier dysfunction, and intractable itch (Weidinger & Novak, 2016). Clinically, H_1-antihistamines are commonly used to treat itch resulting from skin diseases. However, intractable itch in AD is resistant to conventional treatment, such as H_1-antihistamines (Ikoma et al., 2006; Tominaga & Takamori, 2014). Intense itch sensation causes sleep disturbances, depression, and impaired work producibility in AD patients, which reduce quality of life (QOL) (Murota et al., 2010 b; Vakharia et al., 2018).

In the lesional skin of AD, various pruritogens, such as neuropeptides, proteases, cytokines, and opioids, contribute to histamine-independent itch (Paus et al., 2006; Tominaga & Takamori, 2014). These mediators are released from keratinocytes, immune cells, and peripheral nerves (Akiyama & Carstens, 2013). Their receptors (e.g., protease-activated receptor 2 [PAR2], Mas-related G-protein coupled receptors [Mrgprs], and transient receptor potential [TRP] channels) are expressed by itch-mediating C-fibers, and pruritogens activate their specific receptors on sensory C-fibers in skin and transmit itch sensation from the periphery to the central nervous system (Mollanazar et al., 2016; Cevikbas & Lerner, 2020) (Figure 1).

AD patients exhibit increased sensitivity to pruritogenic and non-pruritogenic stimuli such as weak mechanical stimuli (e.g., contact of wool fibers to the skin) (Ikoma et al., 2011). Dysesthesia promotes scratching, which disrupts the skin barrier and exacerbates atopic eczema (Rinaldi, 2019). The itch-scratch cycle is considered to worsen AD symptoms (Otsuka et al., 2017), and, thus, the development of novel therapeutic strategies for intractable itch in AD is needed. In this chapter, we will describe the highlights of recent findings on the mechanisms underlying atopic itch and antipruritic therapies in AD.

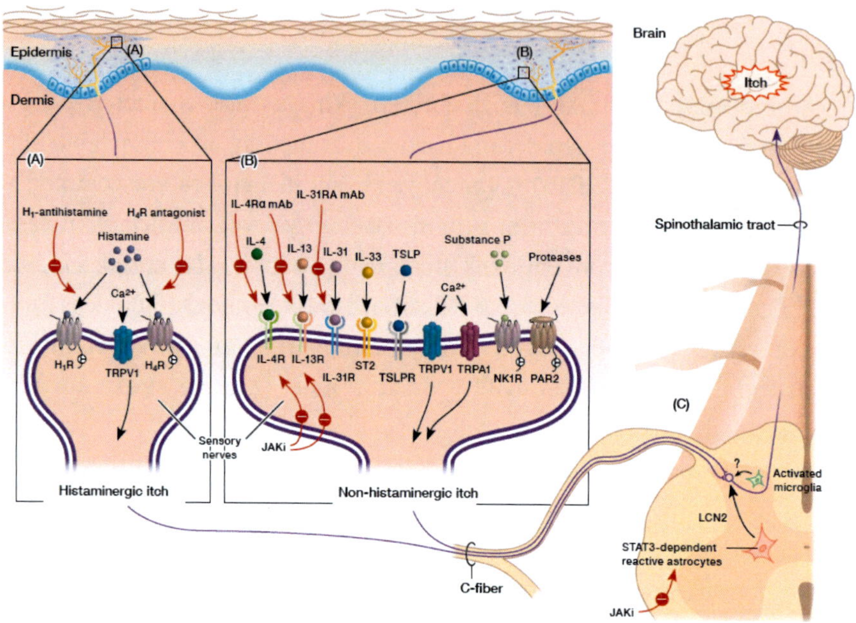

Figure 1. Mechanisms of itch in AD and convincing antipruritic therapies.
Itch in the periphery is categorized as both dependent on (histaminergic) and independent of (non-histaminergic) histamine. Intractable and chronic itch in AD is mainly induced via non-histaminergic pathways. Epidermal nerve fiber density increases in the lesional skin of AD. Pruritus is mediated by various pruritogens binding to pruritoceptors expressed by sensory C-fibers. Peripheral itch signals are transmitted to the brain via $GRPR^+$ neurons in the spinothalamic tract within the spinal cord. (A) Histamine is mainly released from mast cells and binds to receptors, such as H_1R or H_4R. TRPV1 is coupled with histamine receptors and is involved in histaminergic itch. Antihistamines block histamine signaling. (B) Non-histaminergic pruritoceptors require the cation-permeable channels TRPA1 and TRPV1. Various pruritoceptors, such as the cytokine receptors, NK1R and PAR-2, are expressed by non-histaminergic C-fibers and transmit non-histaminergic itch signals. Biologics (e.g., IL-4Rα monoclonal antibody [mAb] and IL-31RA mAb) and JAK inhibitors (JAKi) block cytokine-mediated itch signaling pathways. (C) In the spinal cord, STAT3-dependent reactive astrogliosis is regarded as one of the causes of chronic itch in AD. Lipocalin (LCN) 2 is produced by reactive astrocytes, and enhances GRP-dependent itch signals in the spinal cord. Activated microglia are also considered to play a role in the processing of atopic itch.

2. Mechanisms Underlying Itch in AD

2.1. Skin Barrier and Itch

2.1.1. Skin Barrier

The skin barrier plays a critical role in protecting against the penetration of allergens, pathogens, chemicals, and microbes. This barrier consists of the stratum corneum (SC) and tight junctions (TJs) (Kabashima, 2013). The SC is composed of several layers of corneocytes with intercellular lipid lamellae (e.g., ceramide), a cornified cell envelope (CE), corneodesmosomes, and natural moisturizing factors (NMF) (Cork et al., 2009). Corneocytes are surrounded by an intercellular lipid-enriched matrix, which plays an important role in maintaining skin barrier function and retaining epidermal water (Feingold, 2007; Rawlings & Harding, 2004). The plasma membrane of keratinocytes in the SC replaces the CE with an insoluble protein layer that consists of loricrin, involucrin, filaggrin, and small proline-rich proteins, which are cross-linked by transglutaminases (Candi et al., 2005). This envelope provides strength to corneocytes (Candi et al., 2005; Cork et al., 2009). Corneodesmosomes participate in the cell-cell adhesion of corneocytes and provide physical strength for the SC (Cork et al., 2009; Ishida-Yamamoto & Igawa, 2015). In the SC, filaggrin is rapidly degraded into NMF, including free amino acids and their derivatives, by caspase-14, calpain 1, and bleomycin hydrolase (Kamata et al., 2009). NMF are water-soluble and low-molecular-weight compounds that contribute to the formation of a moisture barrier (Rawlings & Harding, 2004). Corneocytes are constantly shed from the skin surface, which is an important process for maintaining homeostasis in the epidermis. Kallikrein (KLK) family proteases, such as KLK5, 7, and 14, have been shown to contribute to the desquamation process (Cork et al., 2009; Ishida-Yamamoto & Igawa, 2015). TJs are also crucial for the maintenance of skin barrier properties (Tsukita & Furuse, 2002). They are formed at the stratum granulosum (SG2), which comprises cell-cell junctions that seal the intercellular space (Yokouchi et al., 2016).

2.1.2. Skin Barrier Dysfunction in AD

In AD, genetic and environmental factors both play roles in the disruption of the skin barrier (Cork et al., 2009; Weidinger et al., 2018). The measurement of transepidermal water loss (TEWL) is a suitable method for indirectly assessing skin barrier function (Werner & Lindberg, 1985). Previous studies reported that TEWL was increased in the lesional and non-lesional skin of patients with AD (Werner & Lindberg, 1985; Kelleher et al., 2015). These findings suggest that abnormalities in the epidermal barrier are already present in the non-lesional skin of these patients (Lee, 2020).

A loss-of-function mutation in *FLG*, the human gene encoding profilaggrin, is one of the genetic factors causing AD and ichthyoses (Palmer et al., 2006; Sandilands et al., 2009). Although the *FLG* null mutation has been detected in 10-30% of AD patients, the majority of AD patients do not have any *FLG* mutations (Sandilands et al., 2009; Weidinger et al., 2018). The skin barrier is also impaired by exogeneous factors (e.g., soaps and chemicals), allergens (e.g., house dust mites and pollen), infections (e.g., bacteria, such as *Staphylococcus aureus*), and physical stimuli (e.g., scratching, temperature, humidity, and cold dry air) (Hong et al., 2011; Tamagawa-Mineoka & Katoh, 2020). Disruption of the epidermal barrier triggers the release of alarmins, such as thymic stromal lymphopoietin (TSLP) and interleukin (IL)-33 (Trier et al., 2019). These alarmins activate Langerhans cells and initiate Th2 immune responses characterized by IL-4 and IL-13 (Weidinger et al., 2018).

Skin surface pH is elevated in the lesional skin of AD. KLK activity is dependent on pH, and is enhanced when pH in the SC is elevated (Jang et al., 2016). KLK7 is considered to play an important role in the pathogenesis of AD (Kishibe, 2019). KLK7-overexpressing transgenic mice exhibit AD-like symptoms, such as inflammation, severe itch, acanthosis, and hyperkeratosis (Hansson et al., 2002). Furthermore, increases in the expression and chymotryptic activity of KLK7 have been detected in AD lesions (Komatsu et al., 2007; Morizane et al., 2012; Guo et al., 2020). A recent study reported that after the induction of AD, itch behavior was less prominent in KLK7-deficient mice than in wild-type mice (Guo et al., 2020). Thus, KLK7 may be involved in the development of chronic itch in AD.

Granzyme (Gzm) B was recently suggested to impair epidermal barrier function through the cleavage of E-cadherin and filaggrin (Turner et al., 2020). GzmB, a chymase-like serine protease, has been shown to cleave proinflammatory cytokines, such as IL-1α and IL-18, as well as extracellular matrix proteins, including fibronectin and proteoglycans (Susanto et al., 2012; Hiebert & Granville, 2012). GzmB exhibits strong apoptotic activity and plays a role in the pathology of inflammatory skin disease and wound healing (Hussein et al., 2009; Hiebert & Granville, 2012). Plasma GzmB levels were found to be significantly higher in patients with AD than in healthy controls, and correlated with the scoring of atopic dermatitis index (SCORAD), serum severity markers (e.g., thymus and activation-regulated chemokine and lactate dehydrogenase), and itch intensity (Kamata et al., 2016). Furthermore, the plasma concentration of the gastrin-releasing peptide (GRP), an itch-related peptide, correlated with plasma GzmB levels. Therefore, GzmB may play important roles in the induction of barrier dysfunction, inflammation, and itch in AD.

2.1.3. Epidermal Hyperinnevation in Barrier-Disrupted Skin

A correlation has been observed between itch intensity in AD and increases in TEWL (Lee et al., 2006). Histologically, epidermal nerve fiber density was found to be higher in barrier-disrupted skin, such as the lesional skin of AD patients and dry skin model mice, than in normal skin (Tominaga et al., 2007b; Tominaga et al., 2009a). Epidermal hyperinnervation is mainly caused by an imbalance between nerve elongation factors (NEF; e.g., nerve growth factor [NGF] and amphiregulin) and nerve repulsion factors (NRF; e.g., semaphorin 3A [Sema3A] and anosmin-1) (Tominaga & Takamori, 2014), which are produced by keratinocytes in skin.

NGF is an important NEF that promotes skin hyperinnervation (Tominaga & Takamori, 2014). It also up-regulates the expression of neuropeptides, such as substance P (SP) and the calcitonin gene-related peptide (CGRP) (Verge et al., 1995). These neuropeptides are involved in neurogenic inflammation and the hypersensitization of itch sensation (Steinhoff et al., 2003a). A previous study reported that plasma levels of NGF were higher in AD patients than in healthy controls (Toyoda et al., 2002). Similarly, amphiregulin has been shown to play a role in neurite outgrowth as a NEF (Kimura & Schubert, 1992; Nilsson & Kanje, 2005; Tominaga & Takamori, 2014). Its expression was up-regulated in the epidermis of AD model NC/Nga mice (Tominaga et al., 2007a). Furthermore, artemin was found to contribute to cutaneous nerve growth and hypersensitivity to warm sensations in AD (Murota et al., 2012). A recent study reported that mice deficient in the aryl hydrocarbon receptor (AhR), a transcription factor, developed AD-like phenotypes, and air pollutant-activated AhR activated the expression of artemin, alloknesis, epidermal hyperinnervation, and inflammation (Hidaka et al., 2017). The penetration of nerve fibers into the epidermis was attributed to the activation of matrix metalloprotease-2 on the cell surface of growth cones (Tominaga et al., 2009b).

In contrast, Sema3A has been shown to induce the retraction of NGF-responsive sensory afferent neurons (Tang et al., 2004). Semaphorins are a family of secreted and membrane-anchored glycoproteins that act as axon growth cone guidance molecules (Yu & Kolodkin, 1999). Sema3A is one of the best characterized members in this family. It is a secreted molecule that induces growth cone collapse and axon repulsion by interacting with the neuropilin-1/plexin-A1 receptor complex (Tang et al., 2004; Zhou et al., 2008). In normal skin, Sema3A mainly localizes in the suprabasal layers (Tominaga et al., 2008), and its mRNA expression is regulated by the epidermal calcium gradient (Kamata et al., 2020). Epidermal Sema3A levels were previously shown to be lower in the lesional skin of AD than in normal skin (Tominaga et al., 2008). In addition to Sema3A, anosmin-1, an extracellular matrix glycoprotein, inhibited neurite outgrowth in cultured rat dorsal root ganglion (DRG) neurons (Soussi-Yanicostas et al., 1998; Tominaga & Takamori, 2014). It is expressed in the basal layer of the normal epidermis and at lower levels in the lesional skin of AD (Tengara et al., 2010).

Collectively, these findings suggest that decreases in NRF expression levels promote epidermal nerve growth in barrier-disrupted skin, such as AD and xerosis. This epidermal hyperinnervation may increase susceptibility to stimuli and sensitivity to itching. A recent study reported that epidermal nerve fiber density was lower in the lichenified lesions of chronic AD than in healthy skin (Tsutsumi et al., 2016). Furthermore, epidermal hyperinnervation did not contribute to chronic pruritus in the lesional skin of AD (Tan et al., 2019; Pogatzki-Zahn et al., 2020). These discrepancies remain controversial. Although the acute lesions of AD exhibit predominant Th2 polarity, chronic lesions are characterized by the infiltration of both Th1 and Th2 cells (Weidinger & Novak, 2016). The expression of *Sema3A* in cultured normal human epidermal keratinocytes was shown to be up-regulated by the combination of IL-4 and TNF-α or IFN-γ (Kamata et al., 2020). Therefore, these findings suggest that epidermal nerve fiber density varies under different skin conditions in a disease state-dependent manner, such as between the acute and chronic phases.

2.2. Molecular and Cellular Bases of Itch in AD

Chronic pruritus in AD is induced by a histamine-independent pathway (Yosipovitch et al., 2020). Various pruritogen receptors are expressed by histamine-independent (non-histaminergic) C-fiber-innervated skin (Akiyama & Carstens, 2013; Cevikbas & Lerner, 2020). Many different pruritogens, such as histamine, serotonin, protease, and cytokines, activate these receptors (Paus et al., 2006; Yosipovitch et al., 2020) (Figure 1). Itch fibers account for less than 10% of all C-fibers in the skin (Cevikbas & Lerner, 2020). Non-histaminergic pruriceptors require the cation-permeable channels TRPA1 and TRPV1 for itch signaling to the spinal cord (Sun & Dong, 2016; Yosipovitch et al., 2020). Membrane depolarization has been shown to induce the opening of voltage-gated sodium channels, such as Nav 1.7 and Nav 1.8 (Trier et al., 2019; Cevikbas & Lerner, 2020). Itch signals are then rapidly transmitted to the brain via

$GRPR^+$ neurons in the spinothalamic tract within the spinal cord (Akiyama & Carstens, 2013; Yosipovitch et al., 2020).

2.2.1. GRPR

GRP-expressing neurons may mediate the transmission of itch-specific signals from the skin to the central nervous system (Tominaga & Takamori, 2014; Cevikbas & Lerner, 2020). GRP is specifically expressed by DRG neurons, and its receptor GRPR, a G-protein coupled receptor (GPCR) expressed on dorsal spinal cord neurons, specifically transmits itch signals (Sun & Chen, 2007). However, Mishra and Hoon reported that the release of natriuretic peptide precursor B (Nppb [brain natriuretic peptide, BNP]) from DRG neurons induced GRP-GRPR signaling in the spinal cord in response to pruritogens (Mishra & Hoon, 2013). A more recent study showed that GRP^+ neurons in the spinal cord were not required for the transmission of itch signals (Barry et al., 2020). An intrathecal injection of Nppb and GRP significantly increased scratching behavior in mice (Kusube et al., 2016). Furthermore, GRP induced itch behavior more rapidly than Nppb. Thus, although GRP and Nppb play important roles in non-histaminergic itch transmission, Nppb does not appear to be located upstream of GRP.

The density of epidermal nerve fibers containing GRP was previously shown to be increased in AD model NC/Nga mice (Tominaga et al., 2009c). GRP-expressing C- and Aδ fibers in human skin co-express either CGRP or SP (Timmes et al., 2013). Furthermore, serum GRP levels correlated with itch intensity in AD patients (Kagami et al., 2013; Tirado-Sánchez et al., 2015; Kamata et al., 2016). Therefore, serum GRP levels are useful as a marker of itch severity in AD.

2.2.2. Mrgprs

Mrgprs play a role in non-histaminergic itch signaling (Liu et al., 2009; Liu et al., 2011; Sikland et al., 2011; Liu et al., 2012). They are exclusively expressed by neurons in the DRG and trigeminal ganglia (McNeil & Dong, 2014). Mrgprs are divided into subclasses based on sequence homology (Bader et al., 2014; Cevikbas & Lerner, 2020). Mrgpr A3, D, and C11 have been identified on itch-related neurons in mice (Liu et al., 2009; Liu et al., 2011; Liu et al., 2012). An intracutaneous injection of a Mrgpr agonist, such as β-alanine (Mrgpr D agonist), bovine adrenal medulla (BAM) 8-22 (Mrgpr C11 and X1 agonist), or the anti-malaria drug chloroquine (Mrgpr X1 agonist), induced scratching behavior in mice (Han et al., 2002; Lembo et al., 2002; Liu et al., 2009; Sikland et al., 2011; Akiyama et al., 2012; Liu et al., 2012; Ru et al., 2017; Cevikbas & Lerner, 2020). Mrgpr agonist-induced pruritus did not show flares or wheals in the skin (Tominaga & Takamori, 2014). *MrgprA3* mRNA expression levels in the DRG were approximately 2.3-fold higher in AD mice than in control mice (Ko et al., 2016). Also, it has been reported that MrgprB2-deficient mice have decreased pruritus in an allergic contact dermatitis model compared to wild-type mice (Meixiong et al., 2019). These findings suggest that the primary sensory neurons responsive to Mrgpr agonists are part of a non-histaminergic itch neural circuit and a target for treating intractable itch in AD.

2.2.3. PAR-2

PARs belong to the GPCR family. Four PARs, PAR-1 to -4, have been identified by molecular cloning (Vu et al., 1991; Nystedt et al., 1995; Ishihara et al., 1997; Xu et al., 1998). They are activated by a unique mechanism that is dependent on proteolysis. Exogenous and endogenous proteases cleave specific sites within the extracellular N terminus of these receptors (Déry et al., 1998; Macfarlane et al., 2001; Ossovskaya & Bunnett, 2004). The cleavage of PAR-2 is mediated by serine proteases (e.g., KLKs, trypsin, tryptase, prostasin, and matriptase) and also by cysteine proteases (e.g., cathepsin S and the house dust mite antigen Der p1) (Kempkes et al., 2014). This cleavage exposes a new N terminus that acts as a tether ligand, which binds to receptors, thereby activating signaling pathways (Déry et al., 1998; Macfarlane et al., 2001; Ossovskaya & Bunnett, 2004). PAR-2 is widely expressed by a number of cells, such as keratinocytes, endothelial cells, immune cells, and sensory nerve fibers (Bohm et al., 1996; Kempkes et al., 2014). The activation of PAR-2 and -4 by proteases has been shown to induce non-histaminergic itch (Vergnolle et al., 2003; Reddy et al., 2008). PAR-2 levels were found to be elevated in the keratinocytes and skin nerve fibers of AD patients (Steinhoff et al., 2003b; Kempkes et al., 2014). Moreover, a correlation was observed between serum tryptase levels and itch sensation in AD patients (Steinhoff et al., 2003b; Kempkes et al., 2014). Intracutaneous injections of trypsin and tryptase elicited non-histaminergic scratching behavior in mice (Costa et al., 2008; Tsujii et al., 2009; Kempkes et al., 2014). Scratching behavior was suppressed by PAR-2 antagonists or anti-PAR-2 antibodies (Costa et al., 2008; Tsujii et al., 2009; Kempkes et al., 2014). The activation of PAR-2-expressing TRPV1$^+$ nerve fibers was shown to induce the release of CGRP and SP, and promoted itch sensation and neurogenic inflammation (Steinhoff et al., 2003a; Amadesi et al., 2004; Kempkes et al., 2014). In keratinocytes, the activation of PAR-2 has been reported to induce the transcription of TSLP by releasing calcium ions from the endoplasmic reticulum (Wilson et al., 2013a). Secreted TSLP then activates primary afferent neurons and immune cells in the skin (Wilson et al., 2013a). Therefore, PAR-2 may play an important role in non-histaminergic itch in AD, and may be a useful therapeutic target for atopic itch.

2.2.4. TRP Channels

The TRP superfamily consists of non-selective calcium-permeable cation channels. These channels participate in sensory transduction, such as responses to temperature, touch, osmolarity, and nociceptive stimuli (Nilius et al., 2007). TRP channels are expressed in various cells, such as keratinocytes, sensory neurons, immune cells, and melanocytes in the skin (Caterina & Pang, 2016) and comprise six subfamilies: TRPA (ankylin), TRPC (canonical), TRPM (melastatin), TRPML (mucolipin), TRPP (polycystin), and TRPV (vanilloid) (Nilius et al., 2007; Venkatachalam & Montell, 2007). TRPA1, TRPV1, TRPV4, and TRPM8 have been implicated in pruritus (Mollanazar et al., 2016). Furthermore, a recent study demonstrated that TRPV3 contributed to PAR-2-induced pruritus in AD (Zhao et al., 2020).

TRPV1 is expressed by peptidergic nociceptor neurons as well as by keratinocytes and mast cells (Ständer et al., 2004). Its activation has been shown to mediate histaminergic itch (Shim et al., 2007; Kittaka & Tominaga, 2017). However, a topical TRPV1 antagonist (SB705498) failed to exert antipruritic effects on pruritus induced by cowhage or histamine (Gibson et al., 2014). A TRPV1 antagonist (PAC-14028) was previously reported to attenuate dermatitis-associated barrier damage, itch behavior, and inflammation in oxazolone-induced AD model mice (Yun et al., 2011; Lee et al., 2018). A recent study demonstrated that the topical application of 1% PAC-14028 cream significantly reduced visual analogue scale (VAS) itch scores in patients with mild to moderate AD (Lee et al., 2019). Therefore, TRPV1 antagonists may be useful for suppressing atopic itch.

TRPA1 is involved in the transduction of histamine-independent itch from the periphery to the central nervous system (Wilson et al., 2013b; Valdes-Rodriguez et al., 2013). It is expressed on keratinocytes, melanocytes, fibroblasts, and a subpopulation of C-fiber afferents, and is characterized by the co-expression of tropomyosin-related kinase (TrkA) and TRPV1 (Atoyan et al., 2009; Cevikbas & Lerner, 2020). TRPA1 is coupled to MrgprA3 and MrgprC11 on sensory afferents, and its activation induces TRPA1 channel opening (Kittaka & Tominaga, 2017; Cevikbas & Lerner, 2020). Wilson et al. reported that scratching evoked by disruption of the skin barrier was abolished in TRPA1-deficient mice (Wilson et al., 2013b). Furthermore, a topical TRPA1 antagonist (HC030031) blocked skin barrier recovery (Denda et al., 2010).

TRPV4 is expressed by keratinocytes, macrophages, and nociceptive neurons (Kittaka & Tominaga, 2017; Cevikbas & Lerner, 2020). It has been suggested to play an important role in skin barrier recovery and serotonin-induced itch (Kittaka & Tominaga, 2017; Cevikbas & Lerner, 2020). In TRPV4-deficient mice, scratching behavior was attenuated in response to 5-HT, but not to histamine, chloroquine, or SLIGRL (Akiyama et al., 2016). Moreover, a pretreatment with a TRPV4 antagonist (GSK205) inhibited innocuous warming-enhanced serotonin-evoked scratching (Sanders et al., 2018).

TRPM8 is essential for relief from itch and pain by cooling and menthol (Liu & Jordt, 2018; Palkar et al., 2018). It is expressed by sensory neurons that innervate peripheral tissues, such as the skin (McCoy et al., 2011). TRPM8 agonists lead to analgesia (Liu et al., 2013). Similarly, agonists may ameliorate severe itch in dry skin (Ständer et al., 2017).

2.2.5. Neuropeptides and Other Mediators

Histamine is a well-known mediator of acute itch and inflammation. It is mainly released from dermal mast cells and binds to GPCR, such as H_1, H_2, H_3, and H_4 receptors (H_1R, H_2R, H_3R, and H_4R) (Lieberman, 2011). H_1R and H_4R have been identified as pruritoceptors (Simons & Simons, 2011). H_1R is expressed by multiple cell types, such as cells in the nervous system, immune cells, epithelial cells, and endothelial cells, while H_4R is mainly expressed by immune cells (Simons & Simons, 2011). H_1R is linked to the activation of phospholipase A2 and phospholipase C-β3 as well as protein kinase Cδ (Megson et al., 2001; Han et al., 2006; Cevikbas & Lerner, 2020). It mediates histamine-induced increases in vascular permeability and the contraction of airway and vascular smooth muscle cells (Smit et al., 1999). H_1R mediates histaminergic itch associated with urticaria, allergic rhinitis, and allergic conjunctivitis (Simons & Simons, 2011; Thurmond et al., 2014). However, H_1R is not involved in the mechanisms underlying chronic itch in AD (Ikoma et al., 2006; Paus et al., 2006). On the other hand, H_4R has been shown to play a role in the inhibition of adenylate cyclase, and induces the activation of immune cells, such as mast cells, eosinophils, monocytes, dendritic cells, and T cells (Ohsawa & Hirasawa, 2012). Therefore, H_4R may be involved in inflammatory and immune responses involving cytokines in AD (Simons & Simons, 2011; Thurmond et al., 2014).

Neurogenic inflammation is mediated by the release of neuropeptides, such as SP and CGRP (Steinhoff et al., 2003a; Choi & Di Nardo, 2018). In the skin, neuropeptides released from sensory nerve fibers stimulate keratinocytes to produce proinflammatory cytokines (e.g., IL-1α and IL-6) and induce the degranulation of mast cells (Theoharides et al., 1998; Park & Kim, 1999; Song et al., 2000; Steinhoff et al., 2003a). In the periphery, secreted SP has been shown to bind to neurokinin-1 receptors (NK1R) on cutaneous nerve fibers, keratinocytes, and mast cells (Steinhoff et al.,

2003a). In the lesional skin of AD, SP- and CGRP-positive nerve fiber density was increased in the epidermis (Järvikallio et al., 2003; Choi & Di Nardo, 2018). A previous study also reported that serum SP levels were elevated in AD patients and correlated with itch intensity (Salomon & Baran, 2008).

Endothelin (ET)-1 is a peptide that comprises 21 amino acids and is expressed by various cells, such as immune cells, endothelial cells, keratinocytes, neurons, and glial cells (Aktar et al., 2015; Davenport et al., 2016). It is a potent vasoconstrictor and has been shown to induce pain and itch in rodents and humans (Kedzierski &Yanagisawa, 2001; Gomes et al., 2012). Previous studies reported that an intradermal injection of ET-1 induced scratching behavior in BALB/c mice, and ET-1-induced itch was found to be regulated by ET-converting enzyme 1 (McQueen et al., 2007; Kido-Nakahara et al., 2014). ET-1 levels were also shown to be elevated in the lesional skin of AD patients and AD model NC/Nga mice (Kido-Nakahara et al., 2014; Aktar et al., 2015). Thus, ET-1 may play a role in atopic itch.

2.3. Neuroimmune Mechanisms of Itch in AD

Immunologically, atopic eczema is characterized by the infiltration of Th2 cells and Langerhans cells (Weidinger et al., 2018). Intractable itch in AD is caused by interactions between immune cells, keratinocytes, and non-histaminergic C-fibers. Atopic itch-associated cytokines include IL-4, IL-13, IL-31, and TSLP (Mollanazar et al., 2016; Cevikbas & Lerner, 2020). IL-31 and TSLP directly activate non-histaminergic sensory afferents (Wilson et al., 2013a; Cevikbas et al., 2014), while IL-4 increases the responsiveness of sensory neurons to different pruritogens (Oetjen et al., 2017). A recent study reported that IL-33 also played a role in pruritus with AD (Imai, 2019).

2.3.1. IL-31

IL-31 expression levels were shown to be elevated in the skin of AD (Sonkoly et al., 2006). Serum IL-31 levels were higher in AD patients than in healthy controls and correlated with itch intensity (Ezzat et al., 2011). IL-31 bound to the heterodimeric receptor of IL-31 receptor A (IL-31RA) and oncostatin M receptor β-chain (OSMR β) (Cornelissen et al., 2012), which is expressed by immune cells (e.g., dendritic cells, macrophages, eosinophils, and basophils), keratinocytes, and cutaneous sensory nerves (Nakashima et al., 2018). IL-31 activates the Janus kinase (JAK)- signal transducer and activator of transcription (STAT), Ras/extracellular signal-regulated kinase (ERK), and phosphatidylinositol 3-kinase (PI3K)/Akt signal transduction pathways (Cornelissen et al., 2012). Yamamura et al. recently reported that DOCK8 (negative regulator of endothelial PAS domain protein 1 [EPAS1])-deficient mice exhibited AD-like symptoms, such as dermatitis and pruritus, and serum IL-31 levels were markedly higher in knockout mice than in wild-type mice (Yamamura et al., 2017). Therefore, EPAS1, a transcription factor, plays an important role in the production of IL-31 by $CD4^+$ T cells (Yamamura et al., 2017).

IL-31 mediates pruritus by stimulating a subpopulation of $IL\text{-}31RA^+$ and $TRPV1^+$ or $TRPA1^+$ neurons (Cevikbas et al., 2014; Weidinger et al., 2018). An intradermal or intrathecal injection of IL-31 induced scratching behavior in mice, and IL-31-overexpressing transgenic mice developed severe pruritus (Dillon et al., 2004; Cevikbas et al., 2014). Moreover, neurokinin B was released from DRG neurons in response to IL-31 (Sakata et al., 2019). IL-31 has also been shown to promote nerve elongation similar to NGF *in vitro* and *in vivo* (Feld et al., 2016). These findings suggest that IL-31 is a potent pruritogenic cytokine in the skin.

2.3.2. IL-4 and IL-13

Th2 cytokines, such as IL-4 and IL-13, are prominent in AD lesions and promote the production of antigen-specific IgE antibodies and IgE class switching (Sullivan & Silverberg, 2017; Weidinger et al., 2018). These cytokines are mainly produced in $CD4^+$ T cells, as well as basophils, eosinophils, NKT cells, and type 2 innate lymphoid cells (ILC2) (Junttila,

2018). IL-4 binds to IL-4 receptor α (IL-4Rα), and the IL-4/IL-4Rα complex then interacts with the cytokine receptor common subunit γC or IL-13 receptor α1 (IL-13Rα1) (Junttila, 2018; Weidinger et al., 2018). IL-4 binds to the heterodimer of IL-4Rα and IL-13Rα1, which activates JAK1, while IL-13 binds to IL-13Rα1, which activates JAK2 and tyrosine kinase (TYK) 2 (Weidinger et al., 2018). JAK3 interacts with γC (Junttila, 2018). Activated JAK1, JAK2, JAK3, and TYK2 phosphorylate STAT6, and the phosphorylated homodimer of STAT6 then translocates to the nucleus and regulates the expression of various genes (Weidinger et al., 2018). For example, IL-4 and IL-13 have been shown to induce the expression of TSLP in keratinocytes, which may contribute to pruritus in AD (Bogiatzi et al., 2007; Yosipovitch et al., 2020). Furthermore, Th2 cytokines directly stimulate sensory nerves via IL-4Rα and JAK1 (Oetjen et al., 2017). Although these cytokines were found to activate cultured mouse DRG neurons, they did not elicit itch behavior (Cevikbas & Lerner, 2020). IL-4 may enhance the responsiveness of sensory afferents to multiple itch mediators (Oetjen et al., 2017). It currently remains unclear whether IL-13 exerts similar effects to IL-4. IL-4 and IL-13 were recently reported to directly elicit itch behavior in mice (Campion et al., 2019).

IL-4 or IL-13 as well as TGF-β, mechanical stretch, and cancer-derived factors have been shown to induce the expression of periostin, an extracellular matrix protein that binds to the cell surface receptors of integrin family members (Izuhara et al., 2017). Periostin induces the production of TSLP by keratinocytes, which promotes Th2-type immunoresponses (Shiraishi et al., 2012; Masuoka et al., 2012). Serum periostin levels were found to be significantly higher in AD patients than in healthy controls and psoriasis patients, and a positive correlation was observed between its serum levels and disease severity (Kou et al., 2014). Recent studies demonstrated that an intracutaneous injection of periostin induced itch behavior via integrin αVβ3 in mice, dogs, and monkeys, and directly activated sensory afferents in the DRG (Mishra et al., 2020). Accordingly, periostin may be involved in the chronic itch of inflammatory skin diseases, such as AD.

2.3.3. TSLP

TSLP is expressed by various epithelial cells, including keratinocytes, as well as dendritic cells (Zhang & Zhou, 2012). It binds to the heterodimer of the TSLP receptor (TSLPR) and IL-7 receptor α subunit (IL-7Rα), and induces the phosphorylation of STAT5, JAK1, and JAK2 (Pandey et al., 2000; Zhang & Zhou, 2012). TSLP Ɨ was found to be strongly expressed in the lesional skin of AD patients and also by the airway epithelial cells of asthma patients (Soumelis et al., 2002; Ying et al., 2005). Previous studies demonstrated that TSLP induced the release of pruritogenic Th2 cytokines, such as IL-4 and IL-13, and directly stimulated cutaneous sensory nerves to aggravate pruritus (Wilson et al., 2013a; Weidinger et al., 2018). Wilson et al. reported that the calcium signaling pathway is essential for the release of TSLP from keratinocytes, which then directly stimulates TRPA1$^+$ sensory afferents to induce itching (Wilson et al., 2013a).

2.3.4. IL-33

IL-33 belongs to the IL-1 family and is constitutively expressed in the nucleus of endothelial cells, such as keratinocytes, as alarmin (Moussion et al., 2008). In the skin, it is released from epithelial cells, such as keratinocytes, by cellular damage (e.g., mechanical trauma, including scratching, bacteria, and exogenous proteases) (Imai et al., 2013). IL-33 binds to the heterodimer composed of ST2 and the IL-1 receptor accessory protein (IL-1RAcP) on various cells, such as Th2 cells, ILC2, basophils, mast cells, and keratinocytes, and stimulates Th2-type immune responses (Imai, 2019). The IL-33 receptor, ST2 is also expressed by DRG neurons, and IL-33 induces Ca^{2+} influx into DRG neurons through ST2 (Liu et al., 2016). The knockdown of neuronal ST2 expression by an intrathecal injection of siRNA significantly decreased scratching bouts induced by allergic contact dermatitis (Liu et al., 2016). IL-33 is strongly expressed by epidermal keratinocytes in the lesional skin of AD (Savinko et al., 2012; Imai, 2019; Nakamura et al., 2019). In addition, serum IL-33 levels were found to be higher in AD patients than in healthy controls and patients with urticaria or psoriasis (Tamagawa-Mineoka et al., 2014). Imai et al. reported that IL-33 transgenic mice spontaneously developed severe eczema and scratching (Imai et al., 2013). A recent study showed that IL-33 expression levels in SC correlated with itch intensity (Nakamura et al., 2019). Collectively, these findings suggest that IL-33 is a therapeutic target for the chronic itch of AD.

3. TREATMENT OF ITCH IN AD

Table 1. Therapeutic methods for pruritus in AD

	Therapeutic Methods	Mechanisms underlying antipruritic effects
Topical treatments	Emollients/Moisturizers • Heparinoids etc.	•Reduction in epidermal nerve fiber density •Restoration of epidermal barrier dysfunction
	Topical calcineurin inhibitors • Tacrolimus • Pimecrolimus	•Regulation of T-cell activation and proliferation •Block the production of inflammatory cytokines
	Topical glucocorticosteroids	•Suppression of the release of pro-inflammatory cytokines •Attenuation of local inflammation (Indirect antipruritic effect)
Systemic treatments	Oral immunosuppressants 1) Glucocorticosteroids 2) Methotrexate 3) Azathioprine 4) Mycophenolate mofetil	1) Suppression of inflammation (indirect antipruritic effect) 2, 3, 4) No specific studies on anti-pruritic effects
	Oral calcineurin inhibitors • Cyclosporin A	•Regulation of T-cell activation •Inhibition of the production of NF-AT dependent inflammatory cytokines by T cells
	H_1-Antihistamines	•There is no high-level evidence
	Neurotropin	•Reduction in epidermal nerve fiber density
Photo-therapy	• PUVA • NB-UVB	Normalization of expression levels of axon guidance molecules ⇒ Reduction in epidermal nerve fiber density
	• Excimer laser	Reduction in epidermal nerve fiber density (direct effect)
Biologics	Anti-IL-4Rα mAb • Dupilumab	•Bind to IL-4Rα and inhibit interactions with IL-4 or IL-13 •Block the signaling of both IL-4 and IL-13
JAK inhibitors	Topical JAK inhibitors • Delgocitinib • Tofacitinib • Ruxolitinib etc.	•Inhibition of JAK activity •Block the signaling of multiple cytokines

We herein introduce pre-existing and new drugs (including those being developed), with a focus on antipruritic therapies for AD (Figure 1, Tables 1 and 2).

Table 2. New antipruritic approaches for AD

	Therapeutic Methods	Mechanisms underlying antipruritic effects
New antipruritic approaches	Anti-IL-31RA mAb • Nemolizumab	•Bind to IL-31RA and inhibit interactions with IL-31 •Block the signaling of IL-31
	Anti-IL-13 mAb • Tralokinumab	•Bind to IL-13 and inhibit interactions with the receptor •Block the signaling of IL-13
	Anti-TSLP mAb • Tezepelumab	•Bind to TSLP and inhibit interactions with the receptor •Block the signaling of TSLP
	Anti-IL-33 mAb • Etokimab	•Bind to IL-33 and inhibit interactions with the receptor •Block the signaling of IL-33
	Topical PDE4 inhibitors • E6005 • Crisaborole • Difamilast	•Inhibition of PDE4 activity ⇒ Suppress the production of pro-inflammatory cytokines
	μ–opioid receptor antagonists • Naltrexone	•Block the signaling of μ-opioid
	H_4R antagonists • ZPL-3893787 • JNJ-7777120 • JNJ-39758979	•Block inflammatory responses
	NK1R antagonists • Aprepitant, Serlopitant	•Inhibition of substance P
	Anti-NGF therapy • anti-NGF neutralizing antibody • TrkA inhibitor	•Inhibition of NGF signaling ⇒ Reduction in epidermal nerve fiber density
	Recombinant Sema3A replacement therapy	•Reduction in epidermal nerve fiber density
	Minocycline	•Inhibition of microglial activation
	AG490	•Inhibition of the STAT activator JAK2/3
	SVmab1	•Anti-voltage-gated sodium channel Nav1.7-specific antibody ⇒ Block Nav1.7 signaling

3.1. Topical Treatments

Topical treatments, including emollients, topical calcineurin inhibitors (TCIs), and topical corticosteroids, are mainly used to treat intractable itch in patients with mild to moderate AD.

3.1.1. Emollients

Skin barrier abnormalities contribute to the pathogenesis of AD (Cork et al., 2009; Weidinger & Novak, 2016). Topical emollients are useful for maintaining skin barrier intensity and moisture (Weidinger et al., 2018). Emollients consist of saturated or unsaturated hydrocarbons, including fatty acids, cholesterol, squalene, and ceramides (Purnamawati et al., 2017; Weidinger et al., 2018). They soften the skin by supplying lipids to the SC and inhibit the evaporation of water from the skin surface (Purnamawati et al., 2017; Weidinger et al., 2018). The daily application of an emollient from birth has been shown to reduce the risk of AD onset in high-risk infants (Horimukai et al., 2014; Simpson et al., 2014). Furthermore, topical emollients, such as heparinoid creams, reduced epidermal nerve fiber density and epidermal NGF levels more than topical petrolatum in acute dry skin model mice (Kamo et al., 2011a). In dry skin model mice, the topical application of emollients just after barrier disruption markedly reduced epidermal nerve fiber density, whereas delayed application did not affect the number of intraepidermal nerve fibers (Kamo et al., 2011a). These findings suggest that the application of topical emollients to the skin of AD patients more effectively normalizes epidermal hyperinnervation. However, emollients, such as heparinoid creams and petrolatum, did not reduce itch behavior or attenuate atopic eczema in AD model NC/Nga mice (Negi et al., 2012). Thus, emollients may be useful for preventing cutaneous hyperinnervation in AD or dry skin.

3.1.2. TCIs

TCIs, tacrolimus ointment (0.03 and 0.1% strength) and pimecrolimus cream (1% strength), have been shown to attenuate atopic eczema and pruritus (Weidinger & Novak, 2016; Weidinger et al., 2018; Weisshaar et al., 2019). TCIs are anti-inflammatory drugs that inhibit T-cell activation and proliferation and also suppress the release of inflammatory cytokines (Azzi et al., 2013). The potency of 0.1% tacrolimus was found to be similar to that of moderate potency topical corticosteroids (Weidinger & Novak, 2016; Wollenberg et al., 2018a). Previous studies demonstrated that 0.1% tacrolimus more effectively ameliorated AD symptoms than the less potent topical corticosteroids, 1% pimecrolimus cream and 0.03% tacrolimus (Weidinger & Novak, 2016; Wollenberg et al., 2018a; Weisshaar et al., 2019). In AD model mice, the therapeutic efficacy of tacrolimus was shown to be equal to that of clobetasol propionate (the strongest ranking topical corticosteroid), whereas these drugs did not reduce epidermal nerve fiber density (Noguchi et al., 2017). Therefore, epidermal hyperinnervation may not be related to the therapeutic effects of topical tacrolimus and corticosteroids. Furthermore, proactive therapy with the application of tacrolimus twice a week appeared to suppress the relapse of dermatitis (Wollenberg et al., 2018a). TCIs have been reported to cause a burning sensation when initially applied, which may be due to the activation of TRPV1, and this transient burning sensation diminishes after 5-10 days in most cases (Weisshaar et al., 2019).

3.1.3. Topical Glucocorticosteroids

Topical corticosteroids are regarded as an effective form of anti-inflammatory therapy. They activate glucocorticoid receptors, which inhibit the release of proinflammatory cytokines (Elmariah & Lerner, 2011). They are grouped into several classes according to their efficacy in a vasoconstriction assay (Weidinger et al., 2018). Low-potency agents are administered to young children as well as patients with facial lesions and mild skin lesions (Weidinger & Novak, 2016; Weidinger et al., 2018). In randomized control trials, topical corticosteroids attenuated atopic itch more than a vehicle control (Mollanazar et al., 2016). However, their antipruritic efficacy has been attributed to indirect effects via anti-inflammatory activity (Weisshaar et al., 2019).

3.2. Systemic Treatments

3.2.1. Oral Immunosuppressants

Patients with moderate to severe AD may require treatments with systemic immunosuppressants, such as oral glucocorticosteroids, cyclosporin A (CyA), azathioprine, and methotrexate (Mollanazar et al., 2016; Weidinger & Novak, 2016; Eichenfield et al., 2017; Wollenberg et al., 2018b). CyA has been used to treat pruritus in AD patients (Simon & Bieber, 2014; Weisshaar et al., 2019). It has been approved for the short-term treatment of severe refractory AD in many European countries and Japan (Weidinger et al., 2018). Several double-blind controlled studies demonstrated the efficacy of CyA against pruritus in AD (Wahlgren et al., 1990; Simon & Bieber, 2014; Weisshaar et al., 2019). CyA inhibited the activation of T cells, which suppressed the production of IL-2 and other cytokines (Faulds et al., 1993; Liu, 1993; Khattri et al., 2014). The administration of CyA has also been reported to decrease serum levels of IL-31, an itch-related cytokine, in AD patients (Otsuka et al., 2011). In AD model NC/Nga mice, CyA suppressed scratching behavior and epidermal hyperinnervation and also ameliorated skin inflammation (Ko et al., 2016). It also suppressed increases in the expression of IL-31RA in DRG neurons and the number of IL-31$^+$ cells in the dermis of AD model mice (Ko et al., 2016).

Oral glucocorticosteroids as a short-term treatment may effectively suppress severe exacerbations and pruritus in AD (Simon & Bieber, 2014; Weisshaar et al., 2019). However, they are not approved for long-term control due to their potential side effects (Simon & Bieber, 2014; Wollenberg et al., 2018b; Weisshaar et al., 2019).

Azathioprine is a purine analog that is effective for the treatment of severe AD in adult patients (Wollenberg et al., 2018b). The daily use of azathioprine provided relief from chronic pruritus (Maley & Swerlick, 2015; Weisshaar et al., 2019). Methotrexate is a folic acid antagonist that is effective against psoriasis-associated itch (Dawn & Yosipovitch, 2006). It may also provide relief from pruritus in patients with severe AD (Simon & Bieber, 2014; Weisshaar et al., 2019). Azathioprine and methotrexate have both been shown to improve clinical scores, but appear to be less effective than CyA (Weidinger & Novak, 2016).

3.2.2. H_1-Antihistamines

Previous studies demonstrated that non-sedative H_1-antihistamines, such as olopatadine, bepotastine, and fexofenadine, improved dermatitis scores and inhibited itch behavior in AD model mice (Akamatsu et al., 2006; Tanizaki et al., 2008; Murota et al., 2010a; Murota et al., 2014). In addition, bepotastine suppressed the expression of NGF in cultured keratinocytes (Kamata et al., 2018). However, there is currently no high-level evidence for the suppression of itch in AD patients (Weisshaar et al., 2019). Thus, H_1-antihistamine monotherapy has not been approved for atopic itch (Weidinger & Novak, 2016; Wollenberg et al., 2018b; Weisshaar et al., 2019).

3.2.3. Neurotropin

Neurotropin (NTP) is currently used in Japan and China to treat pain. It is a non-protein extract isolated from the inflamed skin of rabbits inoculated with the vaccinia virus (Yoshii et al., 1989). It was previously shown to inhibit NGF-induced neurite outgrowth in DRG neurons and capsaicin-induced SP release *in vitro* (Taneda et al., 2010). In addition, NTP suppressed intraepidermal nerve growth and increased epidermal *Sema3A* mRNA levels in acetone-treated dry skin model mice (Kamo et al., 2013). In Dfb-treated NC/Nga mice, although NTP significantly reduced scratching behavior, it did not attenuate dermatitis (Kamo et al., 2016). These findings suggest that NTP regulates epidermal nerve fiber density by increasing Sema3A levels in the epidermis, resulting in antipruritic effects, and it may also alleviate neurogenic inflammation by inhibiting the release of SP.

3.3. Phototherapy

Ultraviolet (UV)-based therapy (phototherapy) is useful for the treatment of intractable itch in AD. Phototherapy is recommended for AD that is refractory to topical treatments (Eichenfield et al., 2017; Weidinger et al., 2018). Phototherapy for AD utilizes different UV types, such as UVA1 (340-400 nm), broadband-UVB (290-320 nm), narrowband (NB)-UVB (311-313 nm), and an excimer lamp (308 nm) (Garritsen et al., 2014; Rodenbeck et al., 2016). Psoralen UVA (PUVA) and NB-UVB has been shown to suppress epidermal hyperinnervation by normalizing imbalances in the expression levels of axon guidance molecules (e.g., NGF and Sema3A) in the lesional skin of AD patients (Wallengren & Sundler, 2004; Tominaga et al., 2009a; Kamo et al., 2011b). The excimer lamp is the most effective form of phototherapy for intraepidermal nerve fibers (Kamo et al., 2014a). One of the antipruritic mechanisms of action of phototherapy is considered to involve the inhibition of proinflammatory cytokines, such as IL-1 and tumor necrosis factor-α (Steinhoff et al., 2011; Weisshaar et al., 2019). Kurosaki et al. recently reported that excimer lamp irradiation significantly reduced the abundance of *S. aureus*, attenuated dermatitis, and enhanced skin barrier function (Kurosaki et al., 2020).

3.4. Biologics

Correlations have been observed between Th2 cytokine levels (e.g., IL-4 and IL-13) and the severity of AD (Leung & Guttman-Yassky, 2014). Dupilumab is an anti-IL-4Rα monoclonal antibody that inhibits IL-4 and IL-13 signals (Andrews et al., 2006). It also significantly attenuated atopic eczema and suppressed severe pruritus in AD patients (Beck et al., 2014). Furthermore, the blockade of IL-4 and IL-13 signaling by dupilumab inhibited the expression of epidermal proliferation marker proteins and inflammatory mediators, and promoted the expression of epidermal barrier proteins, structural proteins, and lipid metabolism proteins (Hamilton et al., 2014; Gooderham et al., 2018). These findings suggest that atopic skin is normalized by dupilumab. Clinically, dupilumab is used to treat moderate to severe AD in adult patients (Weidinger et al., 2018; Wollenberg et al., 2018b).

3.5. JAK Inhibitors

The JAK and STAT pathways mediate multiple cytokine signals. JAK inhibitors block the signal transduction pathways of a number of cytokines, including IL-2, -4, -6, -10, -12, -22, and -23 as well as interferon (IFN)-α and γ (Solimani et al., 2019). Therefore, these inhibitors are effective in the treatment of inflammatory skin diseases (e.g., AD and psoriasis) and autoimmune diseases (e.g., lupus erythematosus and dermatomyositis) (Solimani et al., 2019). IL-4Rα and JAK1 on sensory nerves have been suggested to contribute to chronic itch (Oetjen et al., 2017). Several JAK inhibitors are currently being developed for the treatment of AD (Solimani et al., 2019). Topical JAK inhibitors, such as delgocitinib (pan JAK inhibitor) and ruxolitinib (JAK1/2 inhibitor), have been shown to attenuate pruritus and disease severity in AD patients (Nakagawa et al., 2019; Kim et al., 2020). Delgocitinib was approved in Japan in 2020. In small open label trials, oral tofacitinib (JAK1/3 inhibitor) ameliorated refractory atopic eczema in patients with moderate to severe AD (Levy et al., 2015; Wollenberg et al., 2018b). Furthermore, randomized trials demonstrated that topical tofacitinib was effective against AD symptoms (Bissonnette et al., 2016). Therefore, JAK inhibitors may be useful for the treatment of moderate to severe pruritus and dermatitis in AD patients.

3.6. New Therapeutic Approaches

3.6.1. New Biologics

Nemolizumab (CIM331), a humanized anti-IL-31RA monoclonal antibody, inhibits IL-31 signaling (Oyama et al., 2018). In randomized, double-blind, placebo-controlled trials, subcutaneous nemolizumab improved pruritus and Eczema Area and Severity Index (EASI) scores (Nemoto et al., 2016a; Ruzicka et al., 2017; Kabashima et al., 2018). Nemolizumab also improved the sleep quality of AD patients (Nakashima et al., 2018). Other trials on AD are currently ongoing with different biologics, such as an anti-IL-13 antibody (tralokinumab), anti-IL-33 antibody (etokimab), and anti-TSLP antibody (tezepelumab) (Wollenberg et al., 2019; Chen et al., 2019; Simpson et al., 2019).

3.6.2. Phosphodiesterase (PDE) 4 Inhibitors

PDEs are cyclic nucleotide cleavage enzymes. The PDE4 isozyme catalyzes the conversion of cyclic adenosine monophosphate (cAMP) to 5'-AMP. It has been shown to regulate the expression of inflammatory cytokines (Yang et al., 2019). PDE activity was found to be elevated in the leukocytes of AD patients, (Hanifin et al., 1992). Furthermore, the topical PDE4 inhibitor, E6005, ameliorated atopic lesions in AD model mice (Ishii et al., 2013). Similarly, E6005 markedly decreased disease severity and itch scores in children with mild to moderate AD, respectively (Nemoto et al., 2016b). In the US, the topical PDE4 inhibitor, crisaborole, has been approved for the treatment of AD (Weidinger et al., 2018). In addition, in randomized, double-blind, placebo-controlled trials, the new topical PDE4 inhibitor, difamilast, was shown to improve various severity scores in AD patients, such as the VAS itch and EASI scores (Saeki et al., 2020). Thus, PDE4 inhibitors have potential as new antipruritic agents in the treatment of AD.

3.6.3. H_4R Antagonists

H_4R plays a role in inflammatory responses (Thurmond, 2015). The oral administration of the H_4R antagonist JNJ-7777120 attenuated itch behavior and skin inflammation in an allergic dermatitis model (Ohsawa & Hirasawa, 2012). The H_4R antagonist JNJ-39758979 also significantly improved the EASI score and attenuated pruritus in AD patients (Murata et al., 2015). Similar findings were obtained for ZPL-3893787 (Werfel et al., 2019). H_4R is considered to be predominant under Th2 conditions (Gutzmer et al., 2009). A previous study reported that H_4R agonists (clobenpropit and 4-methylhistamine) increased the mRNA levels of IL-31, an itch-related cytokine, in peripheral blood mononuclear cells and Th2 cells (Gutzmer et al., 2009). Thus, H_4R may be a new therapeutic target for AD. On the other hand, H_4R antagonists (JNJ-7777120 and JNJ-28307474) did not inhibit scratching behavior or attenuate dermatitis in *Dermatophagoides farinae* body (Dfb)-NC/Nga mice (Kamo et al., 2014b). Although H_4R antagonists suppressed pruritus in allergic dermatitis in a hapten-induced model of NC/Nga mice (e.g., repeated challenges with picryl chloride), they did not exert this effect in a Dfb ointment-induced model (Ohsawa & Hirasawa, 2012; Kamo et al., 2014b). Therefore, histamine may only have a minor role in the pathogenic mechanisms of AD induced by environmental allergens, such as house dust mite.

3.6.4. Others

As discussed above, NGF is one cause of epidermal hyperinnervation, and plasma NGF levels were found to be higher in AD patients than in healthy controls (Toyoda et al., 2002; Tominaga & Takamori, 2014). Therefore, NGF has been assumed to play an important role in the pathogenesis of AD. Epidermal nerve fiber density and dermatitis scores were lower in AD model mice administered an anti-NGF antibody than in those treated with a control antibody; however, scratching behavior was not suppressed (Takano et al., 2005). The binding of NGF to TrkA receptors has been shown to mediate the transduction of NGF signaling. A TrkA inhibitor, AG879 or K252a, significantly attenuated dermatitis and suppressed itch behavior and epidermal hyperinnervation (Takano et al., 2006). Moreover, Sema3A inhibited the NGF-induced sprouting of sensory nerve fibers, and its expression was significantly decreased in the lesional skin of AD (Tominaga & Takamori, 2014). Previous studies reported that the topical application of a recombinant Sema3A protein significantly reduced itch behavior and improved dermatitis scores in AD model NC/Nga mice (Yamaguchi et al., 2008; Negi et al., 2012). These findings suggest that the inhibition of NGF signaling or the application of Sema3A ointment attenuates the symptoms of AD.

Opioid receptors also play an important role in itching (Bigliardi-Qi et al., 2007; Reich & Szepietowski, 2010). The μ-opioid receptor system and endogenous ligands, such as β-endorphins, are involved in chronic skin diseases (e.g., AD) (Bigliardi-Qi et al., 2007; Reich & Szepietowski, 2010). The topical or oral administration of naltrexone, a μ-opioid receptor antagonist, more strongly attenuated pruritus in patients with AD than a placebo (Bigliardi et al., 2007; Malekzad et al., 2009; Ekelem et al., 2019).

As discussed above, SP is released from cutaneous sensory afferents and induces neurogenic inflammation. A correlation has been reported between serum SP levels and itch intensity in AD patients (Salomon & Baran, 2008). The oral administration of aprepitant, a NK1R antagonist, has been reported to suppress itch in AD or prurigo nodularis (Ständer et al., 2010). In recent open randomized trials, oral aprepitant significantly ameliorated itch intensity and disease severity in AD, whereas it did not significant compared with topical treatment alone (Lönndahl et al., 2018). Thus, the antipruritic effects of NK1R antagonists in AD warrant further investigation.

Microglia, astrocytes, and oligodendrocytes are glial cells. An abnormal increase in reactive astrocytes, referred to as astrogliosis, has been reported to cause chronic itch (Shiratori-Hayashi et al., 2015). Shiratori-Hayashi et al. showed that the intrathecal administration of AG490 (inhibitor of STAT3 activator JAK2/3) abolished increases in GRP-evoked scratching in AD model mice (Shiratori-Hayashi et al., 2015). Activated microglia have also been suggested to play a role in atopic itch. Torigoe et al. reported that intrathecal minocycline (inhibitor of activated microglia) suppressed itch behavior and attenuated dermatitis in AD model Dfb-treated NC/Nga mice (Torigoe et al., 2016).

Nav1.7 was shown to play a role in the transmission of pain and itch signals (Cevikbas & Lerner, 2020). Furthermore, Lee et al. demonstrated that the intrathecal or intravenous administration of a Nav1.7-specific antibody (called SVmab1) suppressed spontaneous itch in acetone-diethyl ether and water-induced chronic dry skin model mice (Lee et al., 2014). These new strategies will also be promising for the treatment of atopic itch.

Conclusion

This chapter described the most recent findings on the treatment of pruritus in AD. New drugs that target neural or neuroimmune pathways have been developed for AD. Biologics, such as dupilumab, may be useful for the suppression of inflammation and itching; however, they may not have the capacity to completely suppress intractable itch in AD. New therapeutic drugs, such as JAK inhibitors, may ameliorate severe pruritus. These new therapeutic approaches are required for the treatment of intractable itch and improvements in the QOL of patients with AD. The mechanisms underlying intractable itch in AD are complex, and, thus, require the development of various antipruritic therapies.

Acknowledgments

This work was partly supported by grants from a Research Fellowship from the Japan Society for the Promotion of Science (Grant Number: JP13J09449), JSPS KAKENHI (Grant Numbers: JP15K08680, JP16K08997, JP16K19739, JP18K07396, JP19K08756, and JP20H03568), the Strategic Research Foundation Grant-aided Project for Private Universities from MEXT (Grant Number: S1311011), the Nakatomi Foundation, and the Lydia O'Leary Memorial Foundation.

References

Akamatsu, H., Makiura, M., Yamamoto, N., Yagami, A., Shimizu, Y. and Matsunaga, K. (2006) The effect of fexofenadine on pruritus in a mouse model (HR-ADf) of atopic dermatitis. *J Int Med Res.* 34: 495-504.

Akiyama, T., Tominaga, M., Davoodi, A., Nagamine, M., Blansit, K., Horwitz, A., Carstens, M.I. and Carstens, E. (2012) Cross-sensitization of histamine-independent itch in mouse primary sensory neurons. *Neuroscience* 226: 305-12.

Akiyama, T. and Carstens, E. (2013) Neural processing of itch. *Neuroscience* 250: 697-714.

Akiyama, T., Ivanov, M., Nagamine, M., Davoodi, A., Carstens, M.I., Ikoma, A., Cevikbas, F., Kempkes, C., Buddenkotte, J., Steinhoff, M. and Carstens, E. (2016) Involvement of TRPV4 in Serotonin-Evoked Scratching. *J Invest Dermatol.* 136: 154-160.

Aktar, M.K., Kido-Nakahara, M., Furue, M. and Nakahara, T. (2015) Mutual upregulation of endothelin-1 and IL-25 in atopic dermatitis. *Allergy* 70: 846-54.

Amadesi, S., Nie, J., Vergnolle, N., Cottrell, G.S., Grady, E.F., Trevisani, M., Manni, C., Geppetti, P., McRoberts, J.A., Ennes, H., Davis, J.B., Mayer, E.A. and Bunnett, N.W. (2004) Protease-activated receptor 2 sensitizes the capsaicin receptor transient receptor potential vanilloid receptor 1 to induce hyperalgesia. *J Neurosci.* 24: 4300-12.

Andrews, A.L., Holloway, J.W., Holgate, S.T. and Davies, D.E. (2006) IL-4 receptor alpha is an important modulator of IL-4 and IL-13 receptor binding: implications for the development of therapeutic targets. *J Immunol.* 176: 7456-61.

Atoyan, R., Shander, D. and Botchkareva, N.V. (2009) Non-neuronal expression of transient receptor potential type A1 (TRPA1) in human skin. *J Invest Dermatol.* 129: 2312-5.

Azzi J.R., Sayegh M.H. and Mallat S.G. (2013) Calcineurin inhibitors: 40 years later, can't live without. *J Immunol.* 191: 5785-91.

Bader, M., Alenina, N., Andrade-Navarro, M.A. and Santos, R.A. (2014) Mas and its related G protein-coupled receptors, Mrgprs. *Pharmacol Rev.* 66: 1080-105.

Barry, D.M., Liu, X.T., Liu, B., Liu, X.Y., Gao, F., Zeng, X., Liu, J., Yang, Q., Wilhelm, S., Yin, J., Tao, A. and Chen, Z.F. (2020) Exploration of sensory and spinal neurons expressing gastrin-releasing peptide in itch and pain related behaviors. *Nat Commun.* 11: 1397.

Beck, L.A., Thaçi, D., Hamilton, J.D., Graham, N.M., Bieber, T., Rocklin, R., Ming, J.E., Ren, H., Kao, R., Simpson, E., Ardeleanu, M.,

Weinstein, S.P., Pirozzi, G., Guttman-Yassky, E., Suárez-Fariñas, M., Hager, M.D., Stahl, N., Yancopoulos, G.D. and Radin, A.R. (2014) Dupilumab treatment in adults with moderate-to-severe atopic dermatitis. *N Engl J Med.* 371: 130-9.

Bigliardi-Qi, M., Gaveriaux-Ruff, C., Pfaltz, K., Bady, P., Baumann, T., Rufli, T., Kieffer, B.L. and Bigliardi, P.L. (2007) Deletion of mu- and kappa-opioid receptors in mice changes epidermal hypertrophy, density of peripheral nerve endings, and itch behavior. *J Invest Dermatol.* 127: 1479-88.

Bigliardi, P.L., Stammer, H., Jost, G., Rufli, T., Büchner, S. and Bigliardi-Qi, M. (2007) Treatment of pruritus with topically applied opiate receptor antagonist. *J Am Acad Dermatol.* 56: 979-88.

Bissonnette, R., Papp, K.A., Poulin, Y., Gooderham, M., Raman, M., Mallbris, L., Wang, C., Purohit, V., Mamolo, C., Papacharalambous, J. and Ports, W.C. (2016) Topical tofacitinib for atopic dermatitis: a phase IIa randomized trial. *Br J Dermatol.* 175: 902-911.

Bogiatzi, S.I., Fernandez, I., Bichet, J.C., Marloie-Provost, M.A., Volpe, E., Sastre, X. and Soumelis, V. (2007) Cutting Edge: Proinflammatory and Th2 cytokines synergize to induce thymic stromal lymphopoietin production by human skin keratinocytes. *J Immunol.* 178: 3373-7.

Bohm, S.K., Kong, W., Bromme, D., Smeekens, S.P., Anderson, D.C., Connolly, A., Kahn, M., Nelken, N.A., Coughlin, S.R., Payan, D.G. and Bunnett, N.W. (1996) Molecular cloning, expression and potential functions of the human proteinase-activated receptor-2. *Biochem J.* 314: 1009-16.

Campion, M., Smith, L., Gatault, S., Métais, C., Buddenkotte, J. and Steinhoff, M. (2019) Interleukin-4 and interleukin-13 evoke scratching behaviour in mice. *Exp Dermatol.* 28: 1501-1504.

Candi, E., Schmidt, R. and Melino, G. (2005) The cornified envelope: a model of cell death in the skin. *Nat Rev Mol Cell Biol.* 6: 328-40.

Caterina, M.J. and Pang, Z. (2016) TRP channels in skin biology and pathophysiology. *Pharmaceuticals (Basel).* 9: 77.

Cevikbas, F., Wang, X., Akiyama, T., Kempkes, C., Savinko, T., Antal, A., Kukova, G., Buhl, T., Ikoma, A., Buddenkotte, J., Soumelis, V., Feld,

M., Alenius, H., Dillon, SR., Carstens, E., Homey, B., Basbaum, A. and Steinhoff, M. (2014) A sensory neuron-expressed IL-31 receptor mediates T helper cell-dependent itch: Involvement of TRPV1 and TRPA1. *J Allergy Clin Immunol.* 133: 448-60.

Cevikbas, F. and Lerner, E.A. (2020) Physiology and pathophysiology of itch. *Physiol Rev.* 100: 945-982.

Chen, Y.L., Gutowska-Owsiak, D., Hardman, C.S., Westmoreland, M., MacKenzie, T., Cifuentes, L., Waithe, D., Lloyd-Lavery, A., Marquette, A., Londei, M. and Ogg, G. (2019) Proof-of-concept clinical trial of etokimab shows a key role for IL-33 in atopic dermatitis pathogenesis. *Sci Transl Med.* 11: eaax2945.

Choi, J.E. and Di Nardo, A. (2018) Skin neurogenic inflammation. *Semin Immunopathol.* 40: 249-259.

Cork, M.J., Danby, S.G., Vasilopoulos, Y., Hadgraft, J., Lane, M.E., Moustafa, M., Guy, R.H., Macgowan, A.L., Tazi-Ahnini, R. and Ward, S.J. (2009) Epidermal barrier dysfunction in atopic dermatitis. *J Invest Dermatol.* 129: 1892-908.

Cornelissen, C., Lüscher-Firzlaff, J., Baron, J.M. and Lüscher, B. (2012) Signaling by IL-31 and functional consequences. *Eur J Cell Biol.* 91: 552-66.

Costa, R., Marotta, D.M., Manjavachi, M.N., Fernandes, E.S., Lima-Garcia, J.F., Paszcuk, A.F., Quintão, N.L., Juliano, L., Brain, S.D. and Calixto, J.B. (2008) Evidence for the role of neurogenic inflammation components in trypsin-elicited scratching behaviour in mice. *Br J Pharmacol.* 154: 1094-103.

Davenport, A.P., Hyndman, K.A., Dhaun, N., Southan, C., Kohan, D.E., Pollock, J.S., Pollock, D.M., Webb, D.J. and Maguire, J.J. (2016) Endothelin. *Pharmacol Rev.* 68: 357-418.

Dawn, A. and Yosipovitch, G. (2006) Treating itch in psoriasis. *Dermatol Nurs.* 18: 227-33.

Denda, M., Tsutsumi, M., Goto, M., Ikeyama, K. and Denda, S. (2010) Topical application of TRPA1 agonists and brief cold exposure accelerate skin permeability barrier recovery. *J Invest Dermatol.* 130: 1942-5.

Déry, O., Corvera, C.U., Steinhoff, M. and Bunnett, N.W. (1998) Proteinase-activated receptors: novel mechanisms of signaling by serine proteases. *Am J Physiol.* 274: C1429-52.

Dillon, S.R., Sprecher, C., Hammond, A., Bilsborough, J., Rosenfeld-Franklin, M., Presnell, S.R., Haugen, H.S., Maurer, M., Harder, B., Johnston, J., Bort, S., Mudri, S., Kuijper, J.L., Bukowski, T., Shea, P., Dong, D.L., Dasovich, M., Grant, F.J., Lockwood, L., Levin, S.D., LeCiel, C., Waggie, K., Day, H., Topouzis, S., Kramer, J., Kuestner, R., Chen, Z., Foster, D., Parrish-Novak, J. and Gross, J.A. (2004) Interleukin 31, a cytokine produced by activated T cells, induces dermatitis in mice. *Nat Immunol.* 5: 752-60.

Eichenfield, L.F., Ahluwalia, J., Waldman, A., Borok, J., Udkoff, J. and Boguniewicz, M. (2017) Current guidelines for the evaluation and management of atopic dermatitis: A comparison of the Joint Task Force Practice Parameter and American Academy of Dermatology guidelines *J Allergy Clin Immunol.* 139: S49-S57.

Ekelem, C., Juhasz, M., Khera, P. and Mesinkovska, N.A. (2019) Utility of naltrexone treatment for chronic inflammatory dermatologic conditions: A systematic review. *JAMA Dermatol.* 155: 229-236.

Elmariah, S.B. and Lerner, E.A. (2011) Topical therapies for pruritus. *Semin Cutan Med Surg.* 30: 118-26.

Ezzat, M.H.M, Hasan, Z.E. and Shaheen K.Y.A. (2011) Serum measurement of interleukin-31 (IL-31) in pediatric atopic dermatitis: elevated levels correlate with severity scoring. *J Eur Acad Dermatol Venereol.* 25: 334-9.

Faulds, D., Goa, K.L. and Benfield, P. (1993) Cyclosporin. A review of its pharmacodynamic and pharmacokinetic properties, and therapeutic use in immunoregulatory disorders. *Drugs* 45: 953-1040.

Feingold, K.R. (2007) Thematic review series: skin lipids. The role of epidermal lipids in cutaneous permeability barrier homeostasis. *J Lipid Res.* 48: 2531-46.

Feld, M., Garcia, R., Buddenkotte, J., Katayama, S., Lewis, K., Muirhead, G., Hevezi, P., Plesser, K., Schrumpf, H., Krjutskov, K., Sergeeva, O., Müller, H.W., Tsoka, S., Kere, J., Dillon, S.R., Steinhoff, M. and

Homey, B. (2016) The pruritus- and TH2-associated cytokine IL-31 promotes growth of sensory nerves. *J Allergy Clin Immunol.* 138: 500-508.

Garritsen, F.M., Brouwer, M.W., Limpens, J. and Spuls, P.I. (2014) Photo(chemo)therapy in the management of atopic dermatitis: an updated systematic review with implications for practice and research. *Br J Dermatol.* 170: 501-13.

Gibson, R.A., Robertson, J., Mistry, H., McCallum, S., Fernando, D., Wyres, M. and Yosipovitch, G. (2014) A randomised trial evaluating the effects of the TRPV1 antagonist SB705498 on pruritus induced by histamine, and cowhage challenge in healthy volunteers. *PLoS One.* 9: e100610.

Gomes, L.O., Hara, D.B. and Rae, G.A. (2012) Endothelin-1 induces itch and pain in the mouse cheek model. *Life Sci.* 91: 628-33.

Gooderham, M.J., Hong, H.C., Eshtiaghi, P., Papp, K.A., Gooderham, M.J., Hong, H.C., Eshtiaghi, P., and Papp, K.A. (2018) Dupilumab: A review of its use in the treatment of atopic dermatitis. *J Am Acad Dermatol.* 78 (3 Suppl 1): S28-S36.

Guo, C.J., Mack, M.R., Oetjen, L.K., Trier, A.M., Council, M.L., Pavel, A.B., Guttman-Yassky, E., Kim, B.S. and Liu, Q. (2020) Kallikrein 7 promotes atopic dermatitis-associated itch independently of skin inflammation. *J Invest Dermatol.* 140: 1244-1252.

Gutzmer, R., Mommert, S., Gschwandtner,, M., Zwingmann, K., Stark, H. and Werfel, T. (2009) The histamine H4 receptor is functionally expressed on T(H)2 cells. *J Allergy Clin Immunol.* 123: 619-25.

Hamilton, J.D., Suárez-Fariñas, M., Dhingra, N., Cardinale, I., Li, X., Kostic, A., Ming, J.E., Radin, A.R., Krueger, J.G., Graham, N., Yancopoulos, G.D., Pirozzi, G. and Guttman-Yassky, E. (2014) Dupilumab improves the molecular signature in skin of patients with moderate-to-severe atopic dermatitis. *J Allergy Clin Immunol.* 134: 1293-1300.

Han, S.K., Dong, X., Hwang, J.I., Zylka, M.J., Anderson, D.J. and Simon, M.I. (2002) Orphan G protein-coupled receptors MrgA1 and MrgC11 are distinctively activated by RF-amide-related peptides through the Galpha q/11 pathway. *Proc Natl Acad Sci USA* 99: 14740-5.

Han, S.K., Mancino, V. and Simon, M.I. (2006) Phospholipase Cbeta 3 mediates the scratching response activated by the histamine H_1 receptor on C-fiber nociceptive neurons. *Neuron* 52: 691-703.

Hansson, L., Bäckman, A., Ny, A., Edlund, M., Ekholm, E., Ekstrand Hammarström, B., Törnell, J., Wallbrandt, P., Wennbo, H. and Egelrud, T. (2002) Epidermal overexpression of stratum corneum chymotryptic enzyme in mice: a model for chronic itchy dermatitis. *J Invest Dermatol.* 118: 444-9.

Hanifin, J.M., Lloyd, R., Okubo, K., Guerin, L.L., Fancher, L. and Chan, S.C. (1992) Relationship between increased cyclic AMP-phosphodiesterase activity and abnormal adenylyl cyclase regulation in leukocytes from patients with atopic dermatitis. *J Invest Dermatol.* 98(6 Suppl): 100S-105S.

Hidaka, T., Ogawa, E., Kobayashi, E.H., Suzuki, T., Funayama, R., Nagashima, T., Fujimura, T., Aiba, S., Nakayama, K., Okuyama, R. and Yamamoto, M. (2017) The aryl hydrocarbon receptor AhR links atopic dermatitis and air pollution via induction of the neurotrophic factor artemin. *Nat Immunol.* 18: 64-73.

Hiebert, P.R. and Granville, D.J. (2012) Granzyme B in injury, inflammation, and repair. *Trends Mol Med.* 18: 732-41.

Hong, J., Buddenkotte, J., Berger, T.G. and Steinhoff, M. (2011) Management of itch in atopic dermatitis. *Semin Cutan Med Surg.* 30: 71-86.

Horimukai, K., Morita, K., Narita, M., Kondo, M., Kitazawa, H., Nozaki, M., Shigematsu, Y., Yoshida, K., Niizeki, H., Motomura, K., Sago, H., Takimoto, T., Inoue, E., Kamemura, N., Kido, H., Hisatsune, J., Sugai, M., Murota, H., Katayama, I., Sasaki, T., Amagai, M., Morita, H., Matsuda, A., Matsumoto, K., Saito, H. and Ohya, Y. (2014) Application of moisturizer to neonates prevents development of atopic dermatitis. *J Allergy Clin Immunol.* 134: 824-830.

Hussein, M.R., Abdel-Magid, W.M., Saleh, R. and Nada, E. (2009) Phenotypical characteristics of the immune cells in allergic contact dermatitis, atopic dermatitis and pityriasis rosea. *Pathol Oncol Res.* 15: 73-9.

Ikoma, A., Steinhoff, M., Ständer, S., Yosipovitch, G. and Schmelz, M. (2006) The neurobiology of itch. *Nat Rev Neurosci.* 7: 535-47.

Ikoma, A., Cevikbas, F., Kempkes, C. and Steinhoff, M. (2011) Anatomy and neurophysiology of pruritus. *Semin Cutan Med Surg.* 30: 64-70.

Imai, Y., Yasuda, K., Sakaguchi, Y., Haneda, T., Mizutani, H., Yoshimoto, T., Nakanishi, K. and Yamanishi, K. (2013) Skin-specific expression of IL-33 activates group 2 innate lymphoid cells and elicits atopic dermatitis-like inflammation in mice. *Proc Natl Acad Sci USA* 110: 13921-6.

Imai, Y. (2019) Interleukin-33 in atopic dermatitis. J Dermatol Sci. 96: 2-7.

Ishida-Yamamoto, A. and Igawa, S. (2015) The biology and regulation of corneodesmosomes. *Cell Tissue Res.* 360: 477-82.

Ishihara, H., Connolly, A.J., Zeng, D., Kahn, M.L., Zheng, Y.W., Timmons, C., Tram, T. and Coughlin, S.R. (1997) Protease-activated receptor 3 is a second thrombin receptor in humans. *Nature* 386: 502-6.

Ishii, N., Shirato, M., Wakita, H., Miyazaki, K., Takase, Y., Asano, O., Kusano, K., Yamamoto, E., Inoue, C. and Hishinuma, I. (2013) Antipruritic effect of the topical phosphodiesterase 4 inhibitor E6005 ameliorates skin lesions in a mouse atopic dermatitis model. *J Pharmacol Exp Ther.* 346: 105-12.

Izuhara, K., Nunomura, S., Nanri, Y., Ogawa, M., Ono, J., Mitamura, Y. and Yoshihara, T. (2017) Periostin in inflammation and allergy. *Cell Mol Life Sci.* 74: 4293-4303.

Jang, H., Matsuda, A., Jung, K., Karasawa, K., Matsuda, K., Oida, K., Ishizaka, S., Ahn, G., Amagai, Y., Moon, C., Kim, S.H., Arkwright, P.D., Takamori, K., Matsuda, H. and Tanaka, A. (2016) Skin pH is the master switch of kallikrein 5-mediated skin barrier destruction in a murine atopic dermatitis model. *J Invest Dermatol.* 136: 127-35.

Järvikallio, A., Harvima, I.T. and Naukkarinen, A. (2003) Mast cells, nerves and neuropeptides in atopic dermatitis and nummular eczema. *Arch Dermatol Res.* 295: 2-7.

Junttila, I.S. (2018) Tuning the cytokine responses: An update on interleukin (IL)-4 and IL-13 receptor complexes. *Front Immunol.* 9: 888.

Kabashima, K. (2013) New concept of the pathogenesis of atopic dermatitis: interplay among the barrier, allergy, and pruritus as a trinity. *J Dermatol Sci.* 70: 3-11.

Kabashima, K., Furue, M., Hanifin, J.M., Pulka, G., Wollenberg, A., Galus, R., Etoh, T., Mihara, R., Nakano, M. and Ruzicka, T. (2018) Nemolizumab in patients with moderate-to-severe atopic dermatitis: Randomized, phase II, long-term extension study. *J Allergy Clin Immunol.* 142: 1121-1130.

Kagami, S., Sugaya, M., Suga, H., Morimura, S., Kai, H., Ohmatsu, H., Fujita, H., Tsunemi, Y. and Sato, S. (2013) Serum gastrin-releasing peptide levels correlate with pruritus in patients with atopic dermatitis. *J Invest Dermatol.* 133: 1673-5.

Kamata, Y., Taniguchi, A., Yamamoto, M., Nomura, J., Ishihara, K., Takahara, H., Hibino, T. and Takeda, A. (2009) Neutral cysteine protease bleomycin hydrolase is essential for the breakdown of deiminated filaggrin into amino acids. *J Biol Chem.* 284: 12829-36.

Kamata, Y., Kimura, U., Matsuda, H., Tengara, S., Kamo, A., Umehara, Y., Iizumi, K., Kawasaki, H., Suga, Y., Ogawa, H., Tominaga, M. and Takamori, K. (2016) Relationships among plasma granzyme B level, pruritus and dermatitis in patients with atopic dermatitis. *J Dermatol Sci.* 84: 266-271.

Kamata, Y., Sakaguchi, A., Umehara, Y., Suga, Y., Ogawa, H., Tominaga, M. and Takamori, K. (2018) Bepotastine besilate downregulates the expression of nerve elongation factors in normal human epidermal keratinocytes. *J Dermatol Sci.* 91: 219-231.

Kamata, Y., Tominaga, M., Umehara, Y., Honda, K., Kamo, A., Moniaga, C.S., Komiya, E., Toyama, S., Suga, Y., Ogawa, H. and Takamori, K. (2020) Calcium-inducible MAPK/AP-1 signaling drives semaphorin 3A expression in normal human epidermal keratinocytes. *J Invest Dermatol.* 140:1346-1354.

Kamo, A., Tominaga, M., Negi, O., Tengara, S., Ogawa, H. and Takamori, K. (2011) Topical application of emollients prevents dry skin-inducible intraepidermal nerve growth in acetone-treated mice. *J Dermatol Sci.* 62: 64-6.

Kamo, A., Tominaga, M., Tengara, S., Ogawa, H. and Takamori, K. (2011) Inhibitory effects of UV-based therapy on dry skin-inducible nerve growth in acetone-treated mice. *J Dermatol Sci.* 62: 91-7.

Kamo, A., Tominaga, M., Taneda, K., Ogawa, H. and Takamori, K. (2013) Neurotropin inhibits the increase in intraepidermal nerve density in the acetone-treated dry-skin mouse model. *Clin Exp Dermatol.* 38: 665-8.

Kamo, A., Tominaga, M., Kamata, Y., Kaneda, K., Ko, K.C., Matsuda, H., Kimura, U., Ogawa, H. and Takamori, K. (2014) The excimer lamp induces cutaneous nerve degeneration and reduces scratching in a dry-skin mouse model. *J Invest Dermatol.* 134: 2977-2984.

Kamo, A., Negi, O., Tengara, S., Kamata, Y., Noguchi, A., Ogawa, H., Tominaga, M. and Takamori, K. (2014) Histamine H(4) receptor antagonists ineffective against itch and skin inflammation in atopic dermatitis mouse model. *J Invest Dermatol.* 134: 546-548.

Kamo, A., Tominaga, M., Matsuda, H., Kina, K., Kamata, Y., Umehara, Y., Ogawa, H. and Takamori, K. (2016) Neurotropin suppresses itch-related behavior in NC/Nga mice with atopic dermatitis-like symptoms. *J Dermatol Sci.* 81: 212-5.

Kedzierski, R.M. and Yanagisawa, M. (2001) Endothelin system: the double-edged sword in health and disease. *Annu Rev Pharmacol Toxicol.* 41: 851-76.

Kelleher, M., Dunn-Galvin, A., Hourihane, J.O., Murray, D., Campbell, L.E., McLean, W.H. and Irvine, A.D. (2015) Skin barrier dysfunction measured by transepidermal water loss at 2 days and 2 months predates and predicts atopic dermatitis at 1 year. *J Allergy Clin Immunol.* 135: 930-5.

Kempkes, C., Buddenkotte, J., Cevikbas, F., Buhl, T. and Steinhoff, M. (2014) Role of PAR-2 in neuroimmune communication and itch. In: Carstens, E., Akiyama, T. (eds.), *Itch: Mechanisms and Treatment.* Boca Raton (FL): CRC Press/Taylor & Francis, Chapter 11.

Khattri, S., Shemer, A., Rozenblit, M., Dhingra, N., Czarnowicki, T., Finney, R., Gilleaudeau, P., Sullivan-Whalen, M., Zheng, X., Xu, H., Cardinale, I., de Guzman Strong, C., Gonzalez, J., Suárez-Fariñas, M., Krueger, J.G. and Guttman-Yassky, E. (2014) Cyclosporine in patients with atopic dermatitis modulates activated inflammatory pathways and reverses epidermal pathology. *J Allergy Clin Immunol.* 133: 1626-34.

Kido-Nakahara, M., Buddenkotte, J., Kempkes, C., Ikoma, A., Cevikbas, F., Akiyama, T., Nunes, F., Seeliger, S., Hasdemir, B., Mess, C., Buhl, T., Sulk, M., Müller, F.U., Metze, D., Bunnett, N.W., Bhargava, A., Carstens, E., Furue, M. and Steinhoff, M. (2014) Neural peptidase endothelin-converting enzyme 1 regulates endothelin 1-induced pruritus. *J Clin Invest.* 124: 2683-95.

Kim, B.S., Sun, K., Papp, K., Venturanza, M., Nasir, A. and Kuligowski, M.E. (2020) Effects of ruxolitinib cream on pruritus and quality of life in atopic dermatitis: Results from a phase 2, randomized, dose-ranging, vehicle- and active-controlled study. *J Am Acad Dermatol.* 82: 1305-1313.

Kimura, H. and Schubert, D. (1992) Schwannoma-derived growth factor promotes the neuronal differentiation and survival of PC12 cells. *J Cell Biol.* 116: 777-83.

Kishibe, M. (2019) Physiological and pathological roles of kallikrein-related peptidases in the epidermis. *J Dermatol Sci.* 95: 50-55.

Kittaka, H. and Tominaga, M. (2017) The molecular and cellular mechanisms of itch and the involvement of TRP channels in the peripheral sensory nervous system and skin. *Allergol Int.* 66: 22-30.

Kimura, H. and Schubert, D. (1992) Schwannoma-derived growth factor promotes the neuronal differentiation and survival of PC12 cells. *J Cell Biol.* 116: 777-83.

Ko, K.C., Tominaga, M., Kamata, Y., Umehara, Y., Matsuda, H., Takahashi, N., Kina, K., Ogawa, M., Ogawa, H. and Takamori, K. (2016) Possible antipruritic mechanism of cyclosporine A in atopic dermatitis. *Acta Derm Venereol.* 96: 624-9.

Komatsu, N., Saijoh, K., Kuk, C., Liu, A.C., Khan, S., Shirasaki, F., Takehara, K., Diamandis, E.P. (2007) Human tissue kallikrein expression in the stratum corneum and serum of atopic dermatitis patients. *Exp Dermatol.* 16: 513-9.

Kou, K., Okawa, T., Yamaguchi, Y., Ono, J., Inoue, Y., Kohno, M., Matsukura, S., Kambara, T., Ohta, S., Izuhara, K. and Aihara, M. (2014) Periostin levels correlate with disease severity and chronicity in patients with atopic dermatitis. *Br J Dermatol.* 171: 283-91.

Kurosaki, Y., Tsurumachi, M., Kamata, Y., Tominaga, M., Suga, Y. and Takamori, K. (2020) Effects of 308 nm excimer light treatment on the skin microbiome of atopic dermatitis patients. *Photodermatol Photoimmunol Photomed.* 36: 185-191.

Kusube, F., Tominaga, M., Kawasaki, H., Yamakura, F., Naito, H., Ogawa, H., Tomooka, Y. and Takamori, K. (2016) Electrophysiological properties of brain-natriuretic peptide- and gastrin-releasing peptide-responsive dorsal horn neurons in spinal itch transmission. *Neurosci Lett.* 627: 51-60.

Lee, C.H., Chuang, H.Y., Shih, C.C., Jong, S.B., Chang, C.H. and Yu, H.S. (2006) Transepidermal water loss, serum IgE and beta-endorphin as important and independent biological markers for development of itch intensity in atopic dermatitis. *Br J Dermatol.* 154: 1100-7.

Lee, J.H., Park, C.K., Chen, G., Han, Q., Xie, R.G., Liu, T., Ji, R.R. and Lee, S.Y. (2014) A monoclonal antibody that targets a NaV1.7 channel voltage sensor for pain and itch relief. *Cell* 157: 1393-404.

Lee, J.H., Choi, C.S., Bae, I.H., Choi, J.K., Park, Y.H. and Park, M. (2018) A novel, topical, nonsteroidal, TRPV1 antagonist, PAC-14028 cream improves skin barrier function and exerts anti-inflammatory action through modulating epidermal differentiation markers and suppressing Th2 cytokines in atopic dermatitis. *J Dermatol Sci.* 91: 184-194.

Lee, Y.W., Won, C.H., Jung, K., Nam, H.J., Choi, G., Park, Y.H., Park, M. and Kim, B. (2019) Efficacy and safety of PAC-14028 cream - a novel, topical, nonsteroidal, selective TRPV1 antagonist in patients with mild-to-moderate atopic dermatitis: a phase IIb randomized trial. *Br J Dermatol.* 180: 1030-1038.

Lee, A.Y. (2020) Molecular mechanism of epidermal barrier dysfunction as primary abnormalities. *Int J Mol Sci.* 21: 1194.

Lembo, P.M., Grazzini, E., Groblewski, T., O'Donnell, D., Roy, M.O., Zhang, J., Hoffert, C., Cao, J., Schmidt, R., Pelletier, M., Labarre, M., Gosselin, M., Fortin, Y., Banville, D., Shen. S.H., Ström, P., Payza, K., Dray, A., Walker, P. and Ahmad, S. (2002) Proenkephalin A gene products activate a new family of sensory neuron--specific GPCRs. *Nat Neurosci.* 5: 201-9.

Leung, D.Y. and Guttman-Yassky, E. (2014) Deciphering the complexities of atopic dermatitis: shifting paradigms in treatment approaches. *J Allergy Clin Immunol.* 134: 769-79.

Levy, L.L., Urban, J. and King, B.A. (2015) Treatment of recalcitrant atopic dermatitis with the oral Janus kinase inhibitor tofacitinib citrate. *J Am Acad Dermatol.* 73: 395-9.

Lieberman, P. (2011) The basics of histamine biology. *Ann Allergy Asthma Immunol.* 106: S2-5.

Liu, J. (1993) FK506 and cyclosporin, molecular probes for studying intracellular signal transduction. *Immunol Today* 14: 290-5.

Liu, Q., Tang, Z., Surdenikova, L., Kim, S., Patel, K.N., Kim, A., Ru, F., Guan, Y., Weng, H.J., Geng, Y., Undem, B.J., Kollarik, M., Chen, Z.F., Anderson, D.J. and Dong, X. (2009) Sensory neuron-specific GPCR Mrgprs are itch receptors mediating chloroquine-induced pruritus. *Cell* 139: 1353-65.

Liu, Q., Weng, H.J., Patel, K.N., Tang, Z., Bai, H., Steinhoff, M. and Dong, X. (2011) The distinct roles of two GPCRs, MrgprC11 and PAR2, in itch and hyperalgesia. *Sci Signal.* 4: ra45.

Liu, Q., Sikand, P., Ma, C., Tang, Z., Han, L., Li, Z., Sun, S., LaMotte, R.H. and Dong, X. (2012) Mechanisms of itch evoked by β-alanine. *J Neurosci.* 32: 14532-7.

Liu, B., Fan, L., Balakrishna, S., Sui, A., Morris, J.B. and Jordt, S.E. (2013) TRPM8 is the principal mediator of menthol-induced analgesia of acute and inflammatory. *Pain* 154: 2169-77.

Liu, B., Tai, Y., Achanta, S., Kaelberer, M.M., Caceres, A.I., Shao, X., Fang, J. and Jordt, S.E. (2016) IL-33/ST2 signaling excites sensory neurons and mediates itch response in a mouse model of poison ivy contact allergy. *Proc Natl Acad Sci USA* 113: E7572-E7579.

Liu, B. and Jordt, S.E. (2018) Cooling the itch via TRPM8. *J Invest Dermatol.* 138: 1254-1256.

Lönndahl, L., Holst, M., Bradley, M., Killasli, H., Heilborn, J., Hall, M.A., Theodorsson, E., Holmberg, J. and Nordlind, K. (2018) Substance P antagonist aprepitant shows no additive effect compared with standardized topical treatment alone in patients with atopic dermatitis. *Acta Derm Venereol.* 98: 324-328.

Macfarlane, S.R., Seatter, M.J., Kanke, T., Hunter, G.D. and Plevin, R. (2001) Proteinase-activated receptors. *Pharmacol Rev.* 53: 245-82.

Malekzad, F., Arbabi, M., Mohtasham, N., Toosi, P., Jaberian, M., Mohajer, M., Mohammadi, M.R., Roodsari, M.R. and Nasiri, S. (2009) Efficacy of oral naltrexone on pruritus in atopic eczema: a double-blind, placebo-controlled study. *J Eur Acad Dermatol Venereol.* 23: 948-50.

Maley, A. and Swerlick, R.A. (2015) Azathioprine treatment of intractable pruritus: A retrospective review. *J Am Acad Dermatol.* 73: 439-43.

Masuoka, M., Shiraishi, H., Ohta, S., Suzuki, S., Arima, K., Aoki, S., Toda, S., Inagaki, N., Kurihara, Y., Hayashida, S., Takeuchi, S., Koike, K., Ono, J., Noshiro, H., Furue, M., Conway, S.J., Narisawa, Y. and Izuhara, K. (2012) Periostin promotes chronic allergic inflammation in response to Th2 cytokines. *J Clin Invest.* 122: 2590-600.

McCoy, D.D., Knowlton, W.M. and McKemy, D.D. (2011) Scraping through the ice: Uncovering the role of TRPM8 in cold transduction. *Am J Physiol Regul Integr Comp Physiol.* 300: R1278-87.

McNeil, B. and Dong, X. (2014) Mrgprs as itch receptors. In: Carstens, E. and Akiyama, T. (eds.), *Itch: Mechanisms and Treatment.* Boca Raton (FL): CRC Press/Taylor & Francis, Chapter 12.

McQueen, D.S., Noble, M.A. and Bond, S.M. (2007) Endothelin-1 activates ETA receptors to cause reflex scratching in BALB/c mice. *Br J Pharmacol.* 151: 278-84.

Megson, A.C., Walker, E.M. and Hill, S.J. (2001) Role of protein kinase C alpha in signaling from the histamine H(1) receptor to the nucleus. *Mol Pharmacol.* 59: 1012-21.

Meixiong, J., Anderson, M., Limjunyawong, N., Sabbagh, M.F., Hu, E., Mack, M.R., Oetjen, L.K., Wang, F., Kim, B.S. and Dong, X. (2019) Activation of mast-cell-expressed Mas-related G-protein-coupled receptors drives non-histaminergic itch. *Immunity* 50: 1163-1171.

Mishra, S.K. and Hoon, M.A. (2013) The cells and circuitry for itch responses in mice. *Science.* 340: 968-71.

Mishra, S.K., Wheeler, J.J., Pitake, S., Ding, H., Jiang, C., Fukuyama, T., Paps, J.S., Ralph, P., Coyne, J., Parkington, M., DeBrecht, J., Ehrhardt-Humbert, L.C., Cruse, G.P., Bäumer, W., Ji, R.R., Ko, M.C. and Olivry, T. (2020) Periostin activation of integrin receptors on sensory neurons induces allergic itch. *Cell Rep.* 31: 107472.

Mollanazar, N.K., Smith, P.K. and Yosipovitch, G. (2016) Mediators of chronic pruritus in atopic dermatitis: Getting the itch out? *Clin Rev Allergy Immunol.* 51(3): 263-292.

Morizane, S., Yamasaki, K., Kajita, A., Ikeda, K., Zhan, M., Aoyama, Y., Gallo, R.L. and Iwatsuki, K. (2012) TH2 cytokines increase kallikrein 7 expression and function in patients with atopic dermatitis. *J Allergy Clin Immunol.* 130: 259-61.

Moussion, C., Ortega, N. and Girard, J.P. (2008) The IL-1-like cytokine IL-33 is constitutively expressed in the nucleus of endothelial cells and epithelial cells in vivo: a novel 'alarmin'? *PLoS One* 3: e3331.

Murata, Y., Song, M., Kikuchi, H., Hisamichi, K., Xu, X.L., Greenspan, A., Kato, M., Chiou, C.F., Kato, T., Guzzo, C., Thurmond, R.L., Ohtsuki, M. and Furue, M. (2015) Phase 2a, randomized, double-blind, placebo-controlled, multicenter, parallel-group study of a H4 R-antagonist (JNJ-39758979) in Japanese adults with moderate atopic dermatitis. *J Dermatol.* 42: 129-39.

Murota, H., El-latif, M.A., Tamura, T., Amano, T. and Katayama, I. (2010) Olopatadine hydrochloride improves dermatitis score and inhibits scratch behavior in NC/Nga mice. *Int Arch Allergy Immunol.* 153: 121-32.

Murota, H., Kitaba, S., Tani, M., Wataya-Kaneda, M., Azukizawa, H., Tanemura, A., Umegaki, N., Terao, M., Kotobuki, Y. and Katayama, I. (2010) Impact of sedative and non-sedative antihistamines on the impaired productivity and quality of life in patients with pruritic skin diseases. *Allergol Int.* 59: 345-54.

Murota, H., Izumi, M., Abd El-Latif, M.I., Nishioka, M., Terao, M., Tani, M., Matsui, S., Sano, S. and Katayama, I. (2012) Artemin causes hypersensitivity to warm sensation, mimicking warmth-provoked pruritus in atopic dermatitis. *J Allergy Clin Immunol.* 130: 671-682.

Murota, H., El-latif, M.A., Tamura, T. and Katayama, I. (2014) Olopatadine hydrochloride decreases tissue interleukin-31 levels in an atopic dermatitis mouse model. *Acta Derm Venereol.* 94: 78-9.

Nakagawa, H., Nemoto, O., Igarashi, A., Saeki, H., Oda, M., Kabashima, K. and Nagata, T. (2019) Phase 2 clinical study of delgocitinib ointment in pediatric patients with atopic dermatitis. *J Allergy Clin Immunol.* 144: 1575-1583.

Nakamura, N., Tamagawa-Mineoka, R., Yasuike, R., Masuda, K., Matsunaka, H., Murakami, Y., Yokosawa, E. and Katoh, N. (2019) Stratum corneum interleukin-33 expressions correlate with the degree of lichenification and pruritus in atopic dermatitis lesions. *Clin Immunol.* 201: 1-3.

Nakashima, C., Otsuka, A. and Kabashima, K. (2018) Interleukin-31 and interleukin-31 receptor: New therapeutic targets for atopic dermatitis. *Exp Dermatol.* 27: 327-331.

Negi, O., Tominaga, M., Tengara, S., Kamo, A., Taneda, K., Suga, Y., Ogawa, H. and Takamori, K. (2012) Topically applied semaphorin 3A ointment inhibits scratching behavior and improves skin inflammation in NC/Nga mice with atopic dermatitis. *J Dermatol Sci.* 66: 37-43.

Nemoto, O., Furue, M., Nakagawa, H., Shiramoto, M., Hanada, R., Matsuki, S., Imayama, S., Kato, M., Hasebe, I., Taira, K., Yamamoto, M., Mihara, R., Kabashima, K., Ruzicka, T., Hanifin, J. and Kumagai, Y. (2016) The first trial of CIM331, a humanized antihuman interleukin-31 receptor A antibody, in healthy volunteers and patients with atopic dermatitis to evaluate safety, tolerability and pharmacokinetics of a single dose in a randomized, double-blind, placebo-controlled study. *Br J Dermatol.* 174: 296-304.

Nemoto, O., Hayashi, N., Kitahara, Y., Furue, M., Hojo, S., Nomoto, M. and Shima, S. (2016) Effect of topical phosphodiesterase 4 inhibitor E6005 on Japanese children with atopic dermatitis: Results from a randomized, vehicle-controlled exploratory trial. *J Dermatol.* 43: 881-7.

Nilius, B., Owsianik, G., Voets, T. and Peters, J.A. (2007) Transient receptor potential cation channels in disease. *Physiol Rev.* 87: 165-217.

Nilsson, A. and Kanje, M. (2005) Amphiregulin acts as an autocrine survival factor for adult sensory neurons. *Neuroreport* 16: 213-8.

Noguchi, A., Tominaga, M., Takahashi, N., Matsuda, H., Kamata, Y., Umehara, Y., Ko, K.C., Suga, Y., Ogawa, H. and Takamori, K. (2017) Differences in therapeutic effects of topically applied corticosteroid and tacrolimus on atopic dermatitis-like symptoms in NC/Nga mice. *J Dermatol Sci.* 86: 54-62.

Nystedt, S., Emilsson, K., Larsson, A.K., Strömbeck, B. and Sundelin, J. (1995) Molecular cloning and functional expression of the gene encoding the human proteinase-activated receptor 2. *Eur J Biochem.* 232: 84-9.

Oetjen, L.K., Mack, M.R., Feng, J., Whelan, T.M., Niu, H., Guo, C.J., Chen, S., Trier, A.M., Xu, A.Z., Tripathi, S.V., Luo, J., Gao, X., Yang, L., Hamilton, S.L., Wang, P.L., Brestoff, J.R., Council, M.L., Brasington, R., Schaffer, A., Brombacher, F., Hsieh, C.S., Gereau, R.W. 4th, Miller, M.J., Chen, Z.F., Hu, H., Davidson, S., Liu, Q. and Kim, B.S. (2017) Sensory neurons co-opt classical immune signaling pathways to mediate chronic itch. *Cell* 171: 217-228.

Ohsawa, Y. and Hirasawa, N. (2012) The antagonism of histamine H1 and H4 receptors ameliorates chronic allergic dermatitis via anti-pruritic and anti-inflammatory effects in NC/Nga mice. *Allergy* 67: 1014-22.

Otsuka, A., Nomura, T., Rerknimitr, P., Seidel, J.A., Honda, T. and Kabashima, K. (2017) The interplay between genetic and environmental factors in the pathogenesis of atopic dermatitis. *Immunol Rev.* 278: 246-262.

Otsuka, A., Tanioka, M., Nakagawa, Y., Honda, T., Ikoma, A., Miyachi, Y. and Kabashima, K. (2011) Effects of cyclosporine on pruritus and serum IL-31 levels in patients with atopic dermatitis. *Eur J Dermatol.* 21: 816-7.

Ossovskaya, V.S. and Bunnett, N.W. (2004) Protease-activated receptors: contribution to physiology and disease. *Physiol Rev.* 84: 579-621.

Oyama, S., Kitamura, H., Kuramochi, T., Higuchi, Y., Matsushita, H., Suzuki, T., Goto, M., Adachi, H., Kasutani, K., Sakamoto, A., Iwayanagi, Y., Kaneko, A., Nanami, M., Fujii, E., Esaki, K., Takashima, Y., Shimaoka, S., Hattori, K. and Kawabe, Y. (2018) Cynomolgus monkey model of interleukin-31-induced scratching depicts blockade of human interleukin-31 receptor A by a humanized monoclonal antibody. *Exp Dermatol.* 27: 14-21.

Palkar, R., Ongun, S., Catich, E., Li, N., Borad, N., Sarkisian, A. and McKemy, D.D. (2018) Cooling relief of acute and chronic itch requires TRPM8 channels and neurons. *J Invest Dermatol.* 138: 1391-1399.

Palmer, C.N., Irvine, A.D., Terron-Kwiatkowski, A., Zhao, Y., Liao, H., Lee, S.P., Goudie, D.R., Sandilands, A., Campbell, L.E., Smith, F.J., O'Regan, G.M., Watson, R.M., Cecil, J.E., Bale, S.J., Compton, J.G., DiGiovanna, J.J., Fleckman, P., Lewis-Jones, S., Arseculeratne, G., Sergeant, A., Munro, C.S., El Houate, B., McElreavey, K., Halkjaer, L.B., Bisgaard, H., Mukhopadhyay, S., and McLean, W.H. (2006) Common loss-of-function variants of the epidermal barrier protein filaggrin are a major predisposing factor for atopic dermatitis. *Nat Genet.* 38: 441-6.

Pandey, A., Ozaki, K., Baumann, H., Levin, S.D., Puel, A., Farr, A.G., Ziegler, S.F., Leonard, W.J., Lodish, H.F. (2000) Cloning of a receptor subunit required for signaling by thymic stromal lymphopoietin. *Nat Immunol.* 1: 59-64.

Park, Y.M. and Kim, C.W. (1999) The effects of substance P and vasoactive intestinal peptide on interleukin-6 synthesis in cultured human keratinocytes. *J Dermatol Sci.* 22: 17-23.

Paus, R., Schmelz, M., Bíró, T. and Steinhoff, M. (2006) Frontiers in pruritus research: scratching the brain for more effective itch therapy. *J Clin Invest.* 116: 1174-86.

Pogatzki-Zahn, E.M., Pereira, M.P., Cremer, A., Zeidler, C., Dreyer, T., Riepe, C., Wempe, C., Lotts, T., Segelcke, D., Ringkamp, M., Kremer, A.E., Agelopoulos, K., Ständer, S. (2020) Peripheral sensitization and loss of descending inhibition is a hallmark of chronic pruritus. *J Invest Dermatol.* 140: 203-211.

Purnamawati, S., Indrastuti, N., Danarti, R. and Saefudin, T. (2017) The role of moisturizers in addressing various kinds of dermatitis: A review. *Clin Med Res.* 15: 75-87.

Rawlings, A.V. and Harding, C.R. (2004) Moisturization and skin barrier function. *Dermatol Ther.* 17 (Suppl 1): 43-8.

Reddy, V.B., Iuga, A.O., Shimada, S.G., LaMotte, R.H. and Lerner, E.A. (2008) Cowhage-evoked itch is mediated by a novel cysteine protease: A ligand of protease-activated receptors. *J Neurosci.* 28: 4331-5.

Reich, A. and Szepietowski, J.C. (2010) Opioid-induced pruritus: an update. *Clin Exp Dermatol.* 35: 2-6.

Rinaldi, G. (2019) The itch-scratch cycle: A review of the mechanisms. *Dermatol Pract Concept.* 9: 90-97.

Rodenbeck, D.L., Silverberg, J.I. and Silverberg, N.B. (2016) Phototherapy for atopic dermatitis. *Clin Dermatol.* 34: 607-13.

Ru, F., Sun, H., Jurcakova, D., Herbstsomer, R.A., Meixong, J., Dong, X. and Undem, B.J. (2017) Mechanisms of pruritogen-induced activation of itch nerves in isolated mouse skin. *J Physiol.* 595: 3651-3666.

Ruzicka, T., Hanifin, J.M., Furue, M., Pulka, G., Mlynarczyk, I., Wollenberg, A., Galus, R., Etoh, T., Mihara, R., Yoshida, H., Stewart, J. and Kabashima, K. (2017) Anti-interleukin-31 receptor A antibody for atopic dermatitis. *N Engl J Med.* 376: 826-835.

Saeki, H., Baba, N., Oshiden, K., Abe, Y. and Tsubouchi, H. (2020) Phase 2, randomized, double-blind, placebo-controlled, 4-week study to evaluate the safety and efficacy of OPA- 15406 (difamilast), a new topical selective phosphodiesterase type-4 inhibitor, in Japanese pediatric patients aged 2-14 years with atopic dermatitis. *J Dermatol.* 47: 17-24.

Sakata, D., Uruno, T., Matsubara, K., Andoh, T., Yamamura, K., Magoshi, Y., Kunimura, K., Kamikaseda, Y., Furue, M. and Fukui, Y. (2019)

Selective role of neurokinin B in IL-31-induced itch response in mice. *J Allergy Clin Immunol.* 144: 1130-1133.

Salomon, J. and Baran, E. (2008) The role of selected neuropeptides in pathogenesis of atopic dermatitis. *J Eur Acad Dermatol Venereol.* 22: 223-8.

Sanders, K.M., Hashimoto, T., Sakai, K. and Akiyama, T. (2018) Modulation of Itch by Localized Skin Warming and Cooling. *Acta Derm Venereol.* 98: 855-861.

Sandilands, A., Sutherland, C., Irvine, A.D. and McLean, W.H. (2009) Filaggrin in the frontline: role in skin barrier function and disease. *J Cell Sci.* 122: 1285-94.

Savinko, T., Matikainen, S., Saarialho-Kere, U., Lehto, M., Wang, G., Lehtimäki, S., Karisola, P., Reunala, T., Wolff, H., Lauerma, A. and Alenius, H. (2012) IL-33 and ST2 in atopic dermatitis: expression profiles and modulation by triggering factors. *J Invest Dermatol.* 132: 1392-400.

Shim, W.S., Tak, M.H., Lee, M.H., Kim, M., Kim, M., Koo, J.Y., Lee, C.H., Kim, M. and Oh, U. (2007) TRPV1 mediates histamine-induced itching via the activation of phospholipase A2 and 12-lipoxygenase. *J Neurosci.* 27: 2331-7.

Shiraishi, H., Masuoka, M., Ohta, S., Suzuki, S., Arima, K., Taniguchi, K., Aoki, S., Toda, S., Yoshimoto, T., Inagaki, N., Conway, S.J., Narisawa, Y. and Izuhara, K. (2012) Periostin contributes to the pathogenesis of atopic dermatitis by inducing TSLP production from keratinocytes. *Allergol Int.* 61: 563-72.

Shiratori-Hayashi, M., Koga, K., Tozaki-Saitoh, H., Kohro, Y., Toyonaga, H., Yamaguchi, C., Hasegawa, A., Nakahara, T., Hachisuka, J., Akira, S., Okano, H., Furue, M., Inoue, K. and Tsuda, M. (2015) STAT3-dependent reactive astrogliosis in the spinal dorsal horn underlies chronic itch. *Nat Med.* 21: 927-31.

Sikand, P, Dong, X. and LaMotte, R.H. (2011) BAM8-22 peptide produces itch and nociceptive sensations in humans independent of histamine release. *J Neurosci.* 31: 7563-7.

Simon, D. and Bieber, T. (2014) Systemic therapy for atopic dermatitis. *Allergy* 69: 46-55.

Simons, F.E. and Simons, K.J. (2011) Histamine and H_1-antihistamines: celebrating a century of progress. *J Allergy Clin Immunol.* 128: 1139-1150.

Simpson, E.L., Chalmers, J.R., Hanifin, J.M., Thomas, K.S., Cork, M.J., McLean, W.H., Brown, S.J., Chen, Z., Chen, Y. and Williams, H.C. (2014) Emollient enhancement of the skin barrier from birth offers effective atopic dermatitis prevention. *J Allergy Clin Immunol.* 134: 818-23.

Simpson, E.L., Parnes, J.R., She, D., Crouch, S., Rees, W., Mo, M. and van der Merwe, R. (2019) Tezepelumab, an anti-thymic stromal lymphopoietin monoclonal antibody, in the treatment of moderate to severe atopic dermatitis: A randomized phase 2a clinical trial. *J Am Acad Dermatol.* 80: 1013-1021.

Smit, M.J., Hoffmann, M., Timmerman, H. and Leurs, R. (1999) Molecular properties and signalling pathways of the histamine H1 receptor. *Clin Exp Allergy.* 29: 19-28.

Song, I.S., Bunnett, N.W., Olerud, J.E., Harten, B., Steinhoff, M., Brown, J.R., Sung, K.J., Armstrong, C.A. and Ansel, J.C. (2000) Substance P induction of murine keratinocyte PAM 212 interleukin 1 production is mediated by the neurokinin 2 receptor (NK-2R). *Exp Dermatol.* 9: 42-52.

Sonkoly, E., Muller, A., Lauerma, A.I., Pivarcsi, A., Soto, H., Kemeny, L., Alenius, H., Dieu-Nosjean, M.C., Meller, S., Rieker, J., Steinhoff, M., Hoffmann, T.K., Ruzicka, T., Zlotnik, A. and Homey, B. (2006) IL-31: a new link between T cells and pruritus in atopic skin inflammation. *J Allergy Clin Immunol.* 117: 411-7.

Solimani, F., Meier, K. and Ghoreschi, K. (2019) Emerging topical and systemic JAK inhibitors in dermatology. *Front Immunol.*10: 2847.

Soumelis, V., Reche, P.A., Kanzler, H., Yuan, W., Edward, G., Homey, B., Gilliet, M., Ho, S., Antonenko, S., Lauerma, A., Smith, K., Gorman, D., Zurawski, S., Abrams, J., Menon, S., McClanahan, T., de Waal-Malefyt Rd, R., Bazan, F., Kastelein, R.A. and Liu, Y.J. (2002) Human epithelial cells trigger dendritic cell mediated allergic inflammation by producing TSLP. *Nat Immunol.* 3: 673-80.

Soussi-Yanicostas, N., Faivre-Sarrailh, C., Hardelin, J.P., Levilliers, J., Rougon, G. and Petit, C. (1998) Anosmin-1 underlying the X chromosome-linked Kallmann syndrome is an adhesion molecule that can modulate neurite growth in a cell-type specific manner. *J Cell Sci.* 111: 2953-65.

Ständer, S., Moormann, C., Schumacher, M., Buddenkotte, J., Artuc, M., Shpacovitch, V., Brzoska, T., Lippert, U., Henz, B.M., Luger, T.A., Metze, D. and Steinhoff, M. (2004) Expression of vanilloid receptor subtype 1 in cutaneous sensory nerve fibers, mast cells, and epithelial cells of appendage structures. *Exp Dermatol.* 13: 129-39.

Ständer, S., Siepmann, D., Herrgott, I., Sunderkötter, C. and Luger, T.A. (2010) Targeting the neurokinin receptor 1 with aprepitant: a novel antipruritic strategy. *PLoS One* 5: e10968.

Ständer, S., Augustin, M., Roggenkamp, D., Blome, C., Heitkemper, T., Worthmann, A.C. and Neufang, G. (2017) Novel TRPM8 agonist cooling compound against chronic itch: Results from a randomized, double-blind, controlled, pilot study in dry skin. *J Eur Acad Dermatol Venereol.* 31: 1064-1068.

Steinhoff, M., Ständer, S., Seeliger, S., Ansel J.C., Schmelz, M. and Luger, T. (2003) Modern aspects of cutaneous neurogenic inflammation. *Arch Dermatol.* 139: 1479-88.

Steinhoff, M., Neisius, U., Ikoma, A., Fartasch, M., Heyer, G., Skov, P.S., Luger, T.A. and Schmelz, M. (2003) Proteinase-activated receptor-2 mediates itch: A novel pathway forpruritus in human skin. *J Neurosci.* 23: 6176-80.

Steinhoff, M., Cevikbas, F., Ikoma, A. and Berger, T.G. (2011) Pruritus: management algorithms and experimental therapies. *Semin Cutan Med Surg.* 30: 127-37.

Sun, Y.G. and Chen, Z.F. (2007) A Gastrin-releasing peptide receptor mediates the itch sensation in the spinal cord. *Nature* 448: 700-3.

Sun, S. and Dong, X. (2016) Trp channels and itch. *Semin Immunopathol.* 38: 293-307.

Sullivan, M. and Silverberg, N.B. (2017) Current and emerging concepts in atopic dermatitis pathogenesis. *Clin Dermatol.* 35: 349-353.

Susanto, O., Trapani, J.A. and Brasacchio, D. (2012) Controversies in granzyme biology. *Tissue Antigens* 80: 477-87.

Takano, N., Sakurai, T. and Kurachi, M. (2005) Effects of anti-nerve growth factor antibody on symptoms in the NC/Nga mouse, an atopic dermatitis model. *J Pharmacol Sci.* 99: 277-86.

Takano, N., Sakurai, T., Ohashi, Y. and Kurachi, M. (2007) Effects of high-affinity nerve growth factor receptor inhibitors on symptoms in the NC/Nga mouse atopic dermatitis model. *Br J Dermatol.* 156: 241-6.

Tamagawa-Mineoka, R., Okuzawa, Y., Masuda, K. and Katoh, N. (2014) Increased serum levels of interleukin 33 in patients with atopic dermatitis. *J Am Acad Dermatol.* 70: 882-8.

Tamagawa-Mineoka, R. and Katoh, N. (2020) Atopic dermatitis: Identification and management of complicating factors. *Int J Mol Sci.* 21: 2671.

Tan, Y., Ng, W.J., Lee, S.Z.X., Lee, B.T.K., Nattkemper, L.A., Yosipovitch, G., Ng, L.G. and Tey, H.L. (2019) 3-Dimensional optical clearing and imaging of pruritic atopic dermatitis and psoriasis skin reveals downregulation of epidermal innervation. *J Invest Dermatol.* 139: 1201-1204.

Taneda, K., Tominaga, M., Tengara, S., Ogawa, H. and Takamori, K. (2010) Neurotropin inhibits both capsaicin-induced substance P release and nerve growth factor-induced neurite outgrowth in cultured rat dorsal root ganglion neurones. *Clin Exp Dermatol.* 35: 73-7.

Tang, X.Q., Tanelian, D.L. and Smith, G.M. (2004) Semaphorin3A inhibits nerve growth factor-induced sprouting of nociceptive afferents in adult rat spinal cord. *J Neurosci.* 24: 819-27.

Tanizaki, H., Kambe, N., Nakamura, Y., Tanaka, A., Matsuda, H. and Miyachi, Y. (2008) Oral administration of bepotastine besilate suppressed scratching behavior of atopic dermatitis model NC/Nga mice. *Int Arch Allergy Immunol.* 145: 277-82.

Tengara, S., Tominaga, M., Kamo, A., Taneda, K., Negi, O., Ogawa, H. and Takamori, K. (2010) Keratinocyte-derived anosmin-1, an extracellular glycoprotein encoded by the X-linked Kallmann syndrome gene, is involved in modulation of epidermal nerve density in atopic dermatitis. *J Dermatol Sci.* 58: 64-71.

Theoharides, T.C., Singh, L.K., Boucher, W., Pang, X., Letourneau, R., Webster, E. and Chrousos, G. (1998) Corticotropin-releasing hormone induces skin mast cell degranulation and increased vascular permeability, a possible explanation for its proinflammatory effects. *Endocrinology* 139: 403-13.

Thurmond, R.L., Kazerouni, K., Chaplan, S.R., Greenspan, A.J. (2014) Peripheral neuronal mechanism of itch: histamine and itch. In: Carstens, E. and Akiyama, T. (eds.), *Itch: Mechanisms and Treatment*. Boca Raton (FL): CRC Press/Taylor & Francis, Chapter 10.

Thurmond, R.L. (2015) The histamine H4 receptor: from orphan to the clinic. *Front Pharmacol.* 6: 65.

Timmes, T.R., Rothbaum, R., Kirti, Silva, C.Y., Bhawan, J., Cummins, D.L. and Wolpowitz, D. (2013) Gastrin-releasing peptide-expressing nerves comprise subsets of human cutaneous Aδ and C fibers that may sense pruritus. *J Invest Dermatol.* 133: 2645-2647.

Tirado-Sánchez, A., Bonifaz, A. and Ponce-Olivera, R.M. (2015) Serum gastrin-releasing peptide levels correlate with disease severity and pruritus in patients with atopic dermatitis. *Br J Dermatol.* 173: 298-300.

Tominaga, M., Ozawa, S., Ogawa, H. and Takamori, K. (2007) A hypothetical mechanism of intraepidermal neurite formation in NC/Nga mice with atopic dermatitis. *J Dermatol Sci.* 46: 199-210. a

Tominaga, M., Ozawa, S., Tengara, S., Ogawa, H. and Takamori, K. (2007) Intraepidermal nerve fibers increase in dry skin of acetone-treated mice. *J Dermatol Sci.* 48: 103-11. b

Tominaga, M., Ogawa, H. and Takamori, K. (2008) Decreased production of semaphorin 3A in the lesional skin of atopic dermatitis. *Br J Dermatol.* 158: 842-4.

Tominaga, M., Tengara, S., Kamo, A., Ogawa, H. and Takamori, K. (2009) Psoralen-ultraviolet A therapy alters epidermal Sema3A and NGF levels and modulates epidermal innervation in atopic dermatitis. *J Dermatol Sci.* 55: 40-6.

Tominaga, M., Kamo, A., Tengara, S., Ogawa, H. and Takamori, K. (2009) In vitro model for penetration of sensory nerve fibres on a Matrigel basement membrane: implications for possible application to intractable pruritus. *Br J Dermatol.* 161: 1028-37.

Tominaga, M., Ogawa, H. and Takamori, K. (2009) Histological characterization of cutaneous nerve fibers containing gastrin-releasing peptide in NC/Nga mice: an atopic dermatitis model. *J Invest Dermatol.* 129: 2901-5.

Tominaga, M. and Takamori, K. (2014) Itch and nerve fibers with special reference to atopic dermatitis: therapeutic implications. *J Dermatol.* 41: 205-12.

Torigoe, K., Tominaga, M., Ko, K.C., Takahashi, N., Matsuda, H., Hayashi, R., Ogawa, H. and Takamori, K. (2016) Intrathecal minocycline suppresses itch-related behavior and improves dermatitis in a mouse model of atopic dermatitis. *J Invest Dermatol.* 136: 879-881.

Toyoda, M., Nakamura, M., Makino, T., Hino, T., Kagoura, M and Morohashi, M. (2002) Nerve growth factor and substance P are useful plasma markers of disease activity in atopic dermatitis. *Br J Dermatol.* 147: 71-9.

Trier, A.M., Mack, M.R. and Kim, B.S. (2019) The neuroimmune axis in skin sensation, inflammation, and immunity. *J Immunol.* 202: 2829-2835.

Tsujii, K., Andoh, T., Ui, H., Lee, J.B. and Kuraishi, Y. (2009) Involvement of tryptase and proteinase-activated receptor-2 in spontaneous itch-associated response in mice with atopy-like dermatitis. *J Pharmacol Sci.* 109: 388-95.

Tsukita, S. and Furuse, M. (2002) Claudin-based barrier in simple and stratified cellular sheets. *Curr Opin Cell Biol.* 14: 531-6.

Tsutsumi, M., Kitahata, H., Fukuda, M., Kumamoto, J., Goto, M., Denda, S., Yamasaki, K., Aiba, S., Nagayama, M. and Denda, M. (2016) Numerical and comparative three-dimensional structural analysis of peripheral nerve fibres in epidermis of patients with atopic dermatitis. *Br J Dermatol.* 174: 191-4.

Turner, C.T., Zeglinski, M.R., Richardson, K.C., Santacruz, S., Hiroyasu, S., Wang, C., Zhao, H., Shen, Y., Sehmi, R., Lima, H., Gauvreau, G.M. and Granville, D.J. (2020) Granzyme B contributes to barrier dysfunction in oxazolone-induced skin inflammation through E-cadherin and filaggrin cleavage. *J Invest Dermatol.* In press.

Vakharia, P.P., Cella, D. and Silverberg, J.I. (2018) Patient-reported outcomes and quality of life measures in atopic dermatitis. *Clin Dermatol.* 36: 616-630.

Valdes-Rodriguez, R., Kaushik, S.B. and Yosipovitch, G. (2013) Transient receptor potential channels and dermatological disorders. *Curr Top Med Chem.* 13: 335-43.

Venkatachalam, K. and Montell, C. (2007) TRP Channels. *Annu Rev Biochem.* 76: 387-417.

Verge, V.M., Richardson, P.M., Wiesenfeld-Hallin, Z. and Hökfelt, T. (1995) Differential influence of nerve growth factor on neuropeptide expression in vivo: a novel role in peptide suppression in adult sensory neurons. *J Neurosci.* 15: 2081-96.

Vergnolle, N., Ferazzini, M., D'Andrea, M.R., Buddenkotte, J. and Steinhoff, M. (2003) Proteinase-activated receptors: novel signals for peripheral nerves. *Trends Neurosci.* 26: 496-500.

Vu, T.K., Hung, D.T., Wheaton, V.I. and Coughlin, S.R. (1991) Molecular cloning of a functional thrombin receptor reveals a novel proteolytic mechanism of receptor activation. *Cell* 64: 1057-68.

Wahlgren, C.F., Scheynius, A. and Hägermark, O. (1990) Antipruritic effect of oral cyclosporin A in atopic dermatitis. *Acta Derm Venereol.* 70: 323-9.

Wallengren, J. and Sundler, F. (2004) Phototherapy reduces the number of epidermal and CGRP-positive dermal nerve fibres. *Acta Derm Venereol.* 84: 111-5.

Weidinger, S and Novak, N. (2016) Atopic dermatitis. *Lancet* 387: 1109-1122.

Weidinger, S., Beck, L.A., Bieber, T., Kabashima, K. and Irvine, A.D. (2018) Atopic dermatitis. *Nat Rev Dis Primers* 4: 1.

Weisshaar, E., Szepietowski, J.C., Dalgard, F.J., Garcovich, S., Gieler, U., Giménez-Arnau, A.M., Lambert, J., Leslie, T., Mettang, T., Misery, L., Şavk, E., Streit, M., Tschachler, E., Wallengren, J. and Ständer, S. (2019) European S2k Guideline on Chronic Pruritus. *Acta Derm Venereol.* 99: 469-506.

Werfel, T., Layton, G., Yeadon, M., Whitlock, L., Osterloh, I., Jimenez, P., Liu, W., Lynch, V., Asher, A., Tsianakas, A. and Purkins, L. (2019) Efficacy and safety of the histamine H4 receptor antagonist ZPL-3893787 in patients with atopic dermatitis. *J Allergy Clin Immunol.* 143: 1830-1837.

Werner, Y. and Lindberg, M. (1985) Transepidermal water loss in dry and clinically normal skin in patients with atopic dermatitis. *Acta Derm Venereol.* 65: 102-5.

Wilson, S.R., Thé, L., Batia, L.M., Beattie, K., Katibah, G.E., McClain, S.P., Pellegrino, M., Estandian, D.M. and Bautista, D.M. (2013) The epithelial cell-derived atopic dermatitis cytokine TSLP activates neurons to induce itch. *Cell* 155: 285-95.

Wilson, S.R., Nelson, A.M., Batia, L., Morita, T., Estandian, D., Owens, D.M., Lumpkin, E.A. and Bautista, D.M. (2013) The ion channel TRPA1 is required for chronic itch. *J Neurosci.* 33: 9283-94.

Wollenberg, A., Barbarot, S., Bieber, T., Christen-Zaech, S., Deleuran, M., Fink-Wagner, A., Gieler, U., Girolomoni, G., Lau, S., Muraro, A., Czarnecka-Operacz, M., Schäfer, T., Schmid-Grendelmeier, P., Simon, D., Szalai, Z., Szepietowski, J.C., Taïeb, A., Torrelo, A., Werfel, T. and Ring, J. (2018) Consensus-based European guidelines for treatment of atopic eczema (atopic dermatitis) in adults and children: part I. *J Eur Acad Dermatol Venereol.* 32: 657-682.

Wollenberg, A., Barbarot, S., Bieber, T., Christen-Zaech, S., Deleuran, M., Fink-Wagner, A., Gieler, U., Girolomoni, G., Lau, S., Muraro, A., Czarnecka-Operacz, M., Schäfer, T., Schmid-Grendelmeier, P., Simon,

D., Szalai, Z., Szepietowski, J.C., Taïeb, A., Torrelo, A., Werfel, T. and Ring, J. (2018) Consensus-based European guidelines for treatment of atopic eczema (atopic dermatitis) in adults and children: part II. *J Eur Acad Dermatol Venereol.* 32: 850-878.

Wollenberg, A., Howell, M.D., Guttman-Yassky, E., Silverberg, J.I., Kell, C., Ranade, K., Moate, R. and van der Merwe, R. (2019) Treatment of atopic dermatitis with tralokinumab, an anti-IL-13 mAb. *J Allergy Clin Immunol.* 143: 135-141.

Xu, W.F., Andersen, H., Whitmore, T.E., Presnell, S.R., Yee, D.P., Ching, A., Gilbert, T., Davie, E.W. and Foster, D.C. (1998) Cloning and characterization of human protease-activated receptor 4. *Proc Natl Acad Sci USA* 95: 6642-6.

Yamaguchi, J., Nakamura, F., Aihara, M., Yamashita, N., Usui, H., Hida, T., Takei, K., Nagashima, Y., Ikezawa, Z. and Goshima, Y. (2008) Semaphorin3A alleviates skin lesions and scratching behavior in NC/Nga mice, an atopic dermatitis model. *J Invest Dermatol.* 128: 2842-9.

Yamamura, K., Uruno, T., Shiraishi, A., Tanaka, Y., Ushijima, M., Nakahara, T., Watanabe, M., Kido-Nakahara, M., Tsuge, I., Furue, M. and Fukui, Y. (2017) The transcription factor EPAS1 links DOCK8 deficiency to atopic skin inflammation via IL-31 induction. *Nat Commun.* 8: 13946.

Yang, H., Wang, J., Zhang, X., Zhang, Y., Qin, Z.L., Wang, H. and Luo, X.Y. (2019) Application of topical phosphodiesterase 4 inhibitors in mild to moderate atopic dermatitis: A systematic review and meta-analysis. *JAMA Dermatol.* 155: 585-593.

Ying, S., O'Connor, B., Ratoff, J., Meng, Q., Mallett, K., Cousins, D., Robinson, D., Zhang, G., Zhao, J., Lee, T.H. and Corrigan, C. (2005) Thymic stromal lymphopoietin expression is increased in asthmatic airways and correlates with expression of Th2-attracting chemokines and disease severity. *J Immunol.* 174: 8183-90.

Yoshii, H., Tatsumi, S., Matsuoka, T., Suehiro, S., Konishi, J., Yanagihara, Y., Negoro, S. and Kishimoto, S. (1989) Immunopharmacological actions of an extract isolated from inflamed skin of rabbits inoculated with Vaccinia virus (Neurotropin)--II. Restorative effect on immune responses through the recovery of IL-2 production in aging mice. *Int J Immunopharmacol.* 11: 543-50.

Yosipovitch, G., Berger, T. and Fassett, M.S. (2020) Neuroimmune interactions in chronic itch of atopic dermatitis. *J Eur Acad Dermatol Venereol.* 34: 239-250.

Yu, H.H., Kolodkin, A.L. (1999) Semaphorin signaling: A little less per-plexin. *Neuron* 22: 11-4.

Yun, J.W., Seo, J.A., Jeong, Y.S., Bae, I.H., Jang, W.H., Lee, J., Kim, S.Y., Shin, S.S., Woo, B.Y., Lee, K.W., Lim, K.M. and Park, Y.H. (2011) TRPV1 antagonist can suppress the atopic dermatitis-like symptoms by accelerating skin barrier recovery. *J Dermatol Sci.* 62: 8-15.

Yokouchi, M., Atsugi, T., Logtestijn, M.V., Tanaka, R.J., Kajimura, M., Suematsu, M., Furuse, M., Amagai, M. and Kubo, A. (2016) Epidermal cell turnover across tight junctions based on Kelvin's tetrakaidecahedron cell shape. *elife* 5: e19593.

Yosipovitch, G., Berger, T. and Fassett, M.S. (2020) Neuroimmune interactions in chronic itch of atopic dermatitis. *J Eur Acad Dermatol Venereol.* 34: 239-250.

Zhang, Y. and Zhou, B. (2012) Functions of thymic stromal lymphopoietin in immunity and disease. *Immunol Res.* 52: 211-23.

Zhao, J., Munanairi, A., Liu, X.Y., Zhang, J., Hu, L., Hu, M., Bu, D., Liu, L., Xie, Z., Kim, B.S., Yang, Y. and Chen, Z.F. (2020) PAR2 mediates itch via TRPV3 signaling in keratinocytes. *J Invest Dermatol.* in press doi: 10.1016/j.jid.2020.01.012.

Zhou, Y., Gunput, R.A. and Pasterkamp, R.J. (2008) Semaphorin signaling: progress made and promises ahead. *Trends Biochem Sci.* 33: 161-70.

In: Atopic Dermatitis
Editor: Andreas Maur
ISBN: 978-1-53618-520-1

Chapter 2

COMORBIDITIES IN ATOPIC DERMATITIS

Chanisa Kiatsurayanon[1,2] and François Niyonsaba[3,4]

[1]Institute of Dermatology, Department of Medical Services, Ministry of Public Health, Bangkok, Thailand

[2]Graduate School of Medicine, Rangsit university, Pathumthani, Thailand

[3]Atopy (Allergy) Research Center, Juntendo University Graduate School of Medicine, Tokyo, Japan

[4]Faculty of International Liberal Arts, Juntendo University, Tokyo, Japan

ABSTRACT

Atopic dermatitis is a common chronic inflammatory skin disorder that affects children and adults worldwide. Given the frequent association with elevated serum levels of immunoglobulin E, atopic dermatitis usually encompasses a personal or family history of atopy, which represents a group of disorders including allergic rhinitis, asthma, food allergy and eosinophilic esophagitis. In addition to the well-established knowledge of the relationship between atopic dermatitis and other atopic disorders, increasing evidence has shown that patients with atopic dermatitis also appear to be at higher risk for numerous nonallergic comorbidities, such as infections, neuropsychiatric conditions, metabolic syndrome, cardiovascular diseases, autoimmune diseases and malignancy. Although the pathologic mechanisms behind their links are still largely controversial, these findings suggest cutaneous and systemic immune dysregulation in atopic dermatitis and highlight the possibility that this disease may be more of a systemic disorder than previously perceived. Managing clinicians should be aware of these potential associations and incorporate them into holistic approaches in treating patients with atopic dermatitis. This chapter summarizes the current insight and development in understanding the comorbidities of atopic dermatitis.

Keywords: allergic rhinitis, asthma, atopic dermatitis, cardiovascular disease, innate immunity, mental health disorders, metabolic syndrome, autoimmune disease, malignancy

ABBREVIATIONS

ACD:	allergic contact dermatitis;
AD:	atopic dermatitis;
ADHD:	attention deficit/hyperactivity disorder;
AKC:	atopic keratoconjunctivitis;
AMP:	antimicrobial peptide;
BMI:	body mass index;
CTCL:	cutaneous T cell lymphoma;
CV:	cardiovascular;
DMII:	type 2 diabetes;
hBD:	human β-defensin;
IDA:	iron deficiency anemia;
Ig:	immunoglobulin;
IL:	interleukin;
S. aureus	*Staphylococcus aureus*;
Th:	helper T cell.

1. Introduction

Atopic dermatitis (AD) is a common chronic inflammatory cutaneous disease that affects children and adults of all ages. The impact of AD that reaches beyond the skin and can cause tremendous effects on patients' quality of life has become a global health issue. The association between AD and allergic comorbidities, for example, food allergy, allergic rhinitis, and asthma or so-called 'atopic march', has been well established [1]. Several studies have also addressed the increased risk of allergic contact dermatitis and irritant contact dermatitis among patients with AD [2-4].

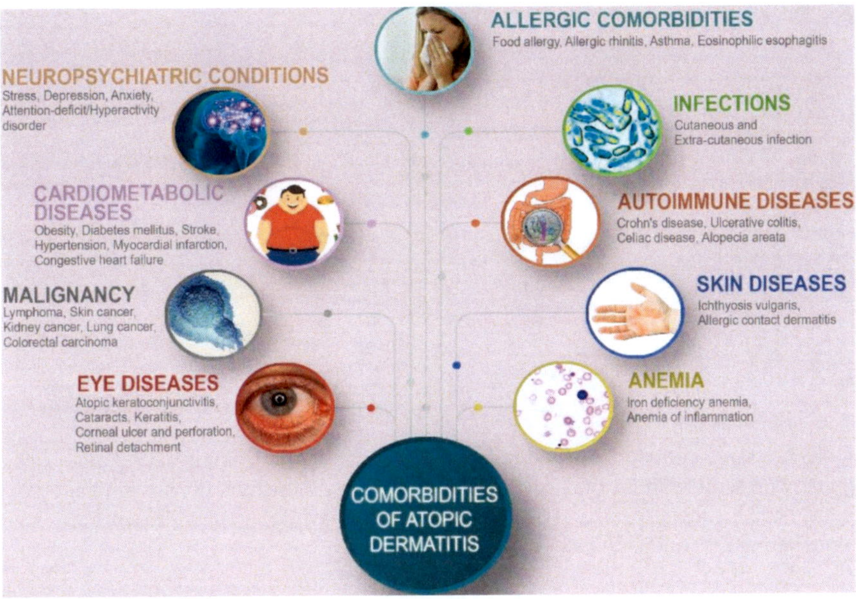

Figure 1. Schematic representation of the comorbidities in atopic dermatitis.

In addition to the well-recognized allergic comorbidities, accumulated evidence has also taken into account the nonallergic comorbidities in patients with AD since AD can be related to other conditions such as neuropsychiatric diseases, obesity, cardiovascular diseases, autoimmune diseases and cancer [1, 5, 6]. Although the full picture behind the mechanisms of these associations is poorly understood, physicians should be aware of this potential coalition to improve treatment outcome and alleviate the burden of disease in patients with AD.

This chapter summarizes the current progress and understanding of the relationship between AD and its comorbidities, which are illustrated in Figure 1. Clinical skin manifestation of AD is shown in Figure 2.

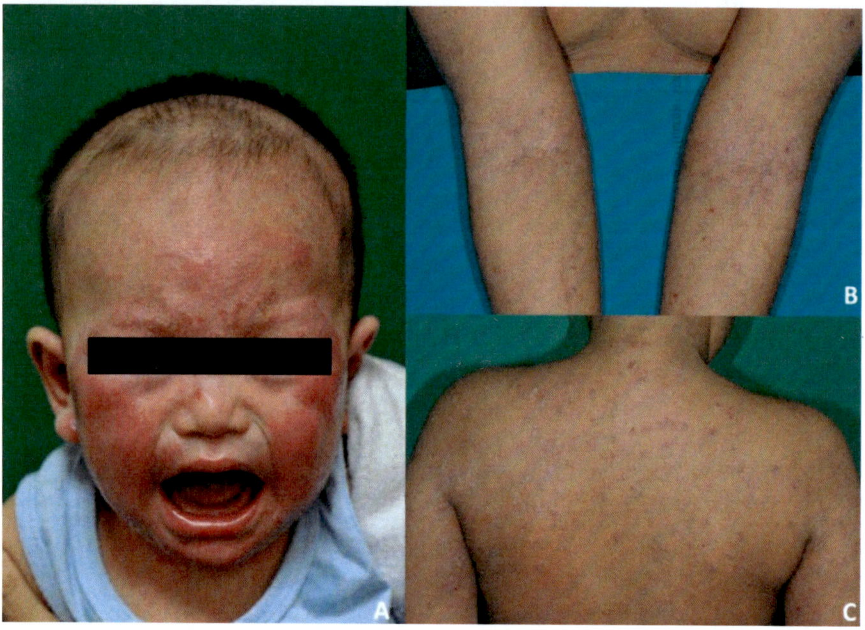

Figure 2. Atopic dermatitis: (A) In infants and young children, atopic dermatitis typically presents with pruritic, erythematous, crusted and scaly lesions prominent on the face and extensor surfaces. (B) and (C) Characteristic flexural and lichenified atopic dermatitis lesions in older children and adults.

2. Comorbidities of AD

2.1. Allergic Comorbidities

Most patients with AD are genetically predisposed to produce abnormal levels of immunoglobulin E (IgE) following exposure to allergens and may develop a typical sequence of other atopic conditions, also called 'atopic march'; for example, food allergy, allergic rhinitis, allergic conjunctivitis, eosinophilic esophagitis and asthma [5, 7-9]. The onset of AD usually begins at a young age. Interestingly, multiple studies indicated that the risk of serial occurrence or progression to atopic march is inversely correlated with the age of onset of AD. Bantz SK et al. demonstrated a significantly higher cumulative incidence of seasonal allergies and asthma among children with AD whose onset was before age 2 when compared to those with AD onset at ages 3 to 7 or 8 to 17 [9]. Likewise, a Canadian cohort study that compared allergic sensitization by skin prick testing in AD and non-AD children at age 1 found a 7-fold increased risk of asthma at age 3 among children in the AD group [10]. In addition, adults with AD are seen to exhibit higher frequencies of developing hand eczema and allergic contact dermatitis, although these conditions are not generally classified as components of atopic march [5, 11, 12]. Patients with AD are also more prone to establish food-induced urticaria/anaphylaxis [13, 14]. Whether there is a causal relationship between AD and the subsequent development of other forms of allergy (i.e., cutaneous, respiratory, food) is still controversial. However, it has been envisaged that epicutaneous sensitization by environmental allergens can occur in the early life of children with AD due to skin barrier defects, thereby increasing the risk of other forms of allergic diseases [15-17]. A United Kingdom study, which investigated children younger than 15 months with a history of AD, found that exposure to peanut antigen in household dust was significantly associated with a 2-fold increased risk of peanut sensitization and peanut allergy later in life [18]. Apart from the inherited skin barrier defect, dysregulation of the innate immune system in patients with AD may further aggravate skin barrier dysfunction through a positive feedback loop [19]. Filaggrin, encoded by the *FLG* gene, is a major protein component of the natural moisturizing factor, which maintains skin hydration and water retention within the stratum corneum. Loss-of-function mutations in the *FLG* gene have been shown to be associated with AD as well as other allergic diseases, including irritant contact dermatitis, asthma, and food allergies [20-22]. Many researchers have documented increased levels of type 2 helper T cells (Th2) and Th22 cytokines (interleukin (IL)-4, IL-13, IL-22 and IL-25) in patients with AD [5]. These cytokines are known to suppress filaggrin expression in keratinocytes and may additionally contribute to barrier defects *in vivo* [23-26].

The essential role of the skin barrier in the development of AD and other allergic diseases has prompted several investigators to explore whether skin barrier enhancement with daily application of emollients could bring about favorable results or halt the development of these diseases [5]. Auspiciously, it was proven that daily application of emollients during the first months of life in neonates decreased the incidence of AD by half and reduced the risk of early allergic sensitization and, therefore, the incidence of respiratory allergies later in life [27-29]. Moreover, recent evidence has demonstrated that application of petrolatum could increase barrier protein and antimicrobial peptide (AMP) expression and decrease proinflammatory cytokines, implying that emollients likely offer more than just skin barrier substitution [30]. Nevertheless, further research is needed to better understand the correlation between atopic diseases and AD and to elucidate the mechanisms behind these associations.

2.2. Neuropsychiatric Conditions

There is a growing body of evidence that neuropsychiatric conditions such as stress, depression, anxiety disorders, attention deficit/hyperactivity disorder and even suicidal ideation are more common in patients with AD than in the general population [31-34]. The association between AD and neuropsychiatric conditions may be attributable to the AD disease severity itself and other factors, such as debilitating pruritus and poor sleep quality, that may negatively affect the patient's quality of life and psychosocial function [32].

Depression is a chronic medical condition characterized by depressed mood, lack of energy, sadness, insomnia, and inability to enjoy life. Other possible accompanying symptoms of depression are sleep disorders, low appetite, decreased ability to concentrate, low self-esteem, feelings of guilt, negative thoughts, suicidal ideation, and suicide attempts [34]. A United States cross-sectional study in 2015 reported a higher prevalence of depression and symptoms related to depression, such as feeling of guilt, loss of energy, poor concentration, and suicidal tendencies, in patients with AD [35]. In addition, moderate and severe forms of AD are significantly more often associated with depression and somatization than mild forms of AD [36]. A study in Germany revealed a higher prevalence of suicidal ideation among patients with AD, especially if they also had depression, severe illness, young age or poor family support [37], which is in parallel with the results from a Korean investigation that reported an increased risk of depressive symptoms, suicidal thoughts and suicidal attempts among adolescent patients with AD [38]. In 2019, a meta-analysis of 37 observational studies found a nearly 2-fold increased risk of depression in patients with AD compared with individuals without AD and that patients with AD were also more likely to have suicidal ideas [39].

In addition to depression, multiple studies worldwide have confirmed the established relationship of AD and anxiety disorders ranging from panic disorder and phobias to generalized anxiety disorder, which can also lead to suicidal ideation [34, 40]. A Danish meta-analysis found a significant association among AD, depression and anxiety and that patients with AD were more likely to be prescribed anxiolytic agents and antidepressants than were controls [40, 41]. Moreover, a large longitudinal cohort study in Taiwan revealed that adolescents and adults with AD are at increased risk of developing major depression, depressive disorders and anxiety disorders later in life when compared to their age- and sex-matched controls [42]. Interestingly, females tend to develop depression and anxiety more than males [43], and emerging evidence has demonstrated that there is a familial aggregation of AD, depression, and anxiety in twins, regardless of their own atopic status [44].

The mechanism behind the contribution of AD to the development of depression and anxiety disorders is still under debate. However, it has been shown that the pathophysiology of depression may be associated with the body's inflammatory responses. Individuals with depression are found to have higher levels of proinflammatory cytokines and acute phase proteins such as IL-4, IL-6, tumor necrosis factor (TNF)-α and C-reactive protein [45]. In contrast, IL-4 deficiency was shown to increase depressive phenotypes in mice, suggesting that IL-4 might be protective against depression [46]. Although IL-4 is a major Th2 cytokine that has the ability to downregulate inflammation, it has been identified as one of the main culprits that drives the development and promotes inflammation in acute AD via a variety of mechanisms; for example, downregulation of filaggrin and AMPs recruits inflammatory cells and causes skin barrier disruption [47]. By blocking multiple cytokine signaling pathways, including IL-4, IL-5 and IL-13, treatment with the Janus kinase (JAK) inhibitors tofacitinib and baricitinib was found to be beneficial in patients with AD [48, 49]. Intriguingly, a phase 3 randomized, placebo-controlled trial recently reported successful treatment of depression and anxiety with the IL-4 receptor antagonist dupilumab [50]. These results imply a plausible molecular link between the pathogenesis of AD, depression, and anxiety.

With regard to attention deficit/hyperactivity disorder (ADHD), several studies have proposed that children with AD have a greater likelihood of developing ADHD [51-55]. Tsai et al. demonstrated that not only AD but also children with other atopic diseases (e.g., asthma, allergic rhinitis, and allergic conjunctivitis) were at increased risk of suffering from ADHD. Moreover, the risk increased with the number of atopic diseases they had [56]. Similarly, Schmitt et al. also observed a significant association between ADHD and AD regardless of age, sex and other psychiatric conditions, and the risk of developing ADHD increased with each doctor's visit [57]. A prospective cohort study revealed that antihistamine use in early childhood may increase the risk of developing ADHD later in life, but the severity of AD was not correlated with the severity of ADHD symptoms [58]. Furthermore, children with AD were also at a greater risk of exhibiting other behavioral disorders and autism [51, 59]. Interestingly, the risk of developing mental problems corresponds with the duration of having AD [60]. The mechanisms behind the relationship between ADHD and AD are still undiscovered. Some investigators postulated that sleep disturbance secondary to nocturnal pruritus in AD, psychological stress, and dysfunctional neuroinflammatory cytokines in the brain may explain this association [61-63].

Regarding schizophrenia, only a few studies have addressed its association with AD, and the data are still controversial [34]. Pedersen et al. demonstrated that the presence of AD, urticaria, allergic rhinitis or asthma significantly increased the risk of schizophrenia [64]. On the other hand, Okusaga et al. reported a lower level of specific IgE antibodies and a lower prevalence of AD among patients with schizophrenia [65].

For other neuropsychiatric disorders, such as anorexia nervosa, conduct disorder, conversion disorder, and obsessive-compulsive disorder, there is still scant information to confirm their associations with AD, and the results have not been uniformly reproduced [1, 66, 67]. In brief, accumulated evidence strongly supports an established association between AD and certain neuropsychiatric conditions. Clinicians taking care of patients with AD should be vigilant for potential depressive symptoms and other neuropsychiatric manifestations, especially for patients with moderate-to-severe disease who may need psychiatric consultation.

2.3. Infections

It is now widely accepted that AD is strongly correlated with cutaneous *Staphylococcus aureus (S. aureus)* colonization and that the severity of AD lesions is associated with the relative level of *S. aureus* on the skin [1, 68, 69]. An increased number of *S. aureus* and decreased microbial diversity on the skin are detected in AD flares [70]. *S. aureus* was shown to cause skin inflammation in AD directly from the staphylococcal enterotoxin and might even result in systemic immune aberrations such as food allergies [1, 5]. In fact, the prevalence of certain infectious diseases was found to be significantly higher in individuals with AD [1]. A large United States national cohort study found a higher frequency of various types of infections, including systemic infections, in hospitalized patients with AD than in patients without AD [71]. According to multiple studies, patients with AD are more susceptible to both cutaneous and extracutaneous infections. For cutaneous infections, evidence has demonstrated that patients with AD are at a higher risk of getting impetigo, warts, eczema herpeticum, eczema coxsackium, chicken pox and molluscum contagiosum [72-78]. Moreover, patients with AD are at greater risk of extracutaneous infections, including respiratory tract, gastrointestinal and urinary tract infections [76, 77, 79-83]. Recent studies also reported the association of AD and infective endocarditis [84, 85]. Interestingly, the risk of infectious diseases increases with the number of allergic diseases a person has [73].

One of the reasons why patients with AD are more susceptible to certain viral and bacterial infections may be due to skin barrier defects. The epidermis acts as the first line of defense between the body and the environment, keeping environmental antigens, irritants, and microbes from entering while preserving water loss from the body. Since filaggrin, along with other skin barrier-related proteins and enzymes, is genetically defective, the epidermis of individuals with AD might facilitate microbial colonization and invasion [86-88]. Nonetheless, the observation that the skin of patients with psoriasis, which is associated with a comparable degree of epidermal barrier impairment, does not demonstrate a similar propensity for infection as that of patients with AD implies that other factors may presumably contribute to AD pathogenesis [89, 90]. In addition to the skin barrier defect, the dysregulated immune system plus microbiome dysbiosis in AD may further increase the susceptibility to infection. Unlike Th1-mediated inflammation in psoriasis, the pathogenesis of AD is naturally driven by the Th2 inflammatory milieu. Indeed, the decreased Th1/Th2 ratio and increased level of Th2 cytokines, including IL-4, IL-10 and IL-13, are known to inhibit the production of AMPs, including human β-defensin (hBD)-2, hBD-3, cathelicidin LL-37, and dermcidin in AD skin [91-94]. The lower amounts of AMPs in patients with AD than in patients with psoriasis may explain the higher incidence of skin infections in the AD group [95]. Interestingly, a recent finding reported that filaggrin deficiency significantly promoted cutaneous hBD-2 expression, implying a possible compensatory mechanism to ameliorate the skin antimicrobial barrier in a filaggrin-deficient state [96]. In addition, the

Th2 inflammatory environment also promotes cutaneous expression of fibronectin and/or fibrinogen, leading to greater attachment of *S. aureus* to the skin of individuals with AD [97].

Moreover, Th-2-mediated alterations in AMP expression might be implicated in microbiome dysbiosis in AD. Recently, investigators have observed microbiome shifts and a reduction in commensal organisms in AD flares compared with baseline and post flares [70, 98]. Experiments in mice demonstrated improved AD severity with increasing microbial diversity [99], and the skin commensal *Staphylococcus epidermidis* could produce antimicrobial products against bacterial skin infections [100-102]. Furthermore, treatment of AD with nonpathogenic skin commensal bacteria has shown the potential to alleviate cutaneous inflammatory reactions by rebalancing immunological signals. There is evidence that application of extracts from gram-negative bacterium *Vitreoscilla filiformis* lysate could help to restore skin microbial imbalance and potentially improve AD lesions [103]. Modulation of the skin microbiota by application of coal tar induced AMP expression, decreased *Staphylococcus* abundance, and increased *Propionibacterium* affluence, suggesting a shift in microbiome composition towards that of healthy controls, which may reduce AD severity [69]. However, definitive proof of the relationship between the skin microbiota and AD is still missing, and further investigations are required.

Apart from the abovementioned factors, low vitamin D levels, exposure to cigarette smoke and other air pollutants may also contribute to the increased risk of infection observed in patients with AD [104-107].

2.4. Cardiometabolic Diseases: Cardiovascular Diseases, Stroke, Obesity, and Metabolic Syndrome

The relationship between AD and cardiovascular (CV) disease is ambiguous, and previous studies have provided conflicting results. A 2017 systematic review and meta-analysis evaluating the association with CV disease and type 2 diabetes (DMII) in adults with AD did not find an association between AD and DMII, myocardial infarction, stroke or hypertension but found a significantly increased risk of angina pectoris by 50% [108]. Meta-analysis of adjusted data demonstrated similar results. On the other hand, a large population-based cohort study from the United Kingdom comparing adult patients with AD with their age- and sex-matched controls revealed that patients with AD, in particular those with severe disease (as defined by treatment with systemic immunosuppr-essants, phototherapy, or specialist referral), had an increased prevalence of CV diseases, including myocardial infarction, unstable angina, heart failure, atrial fibrillation, and CV death [109]. Emerging evidence suggests that adults with AD also tend to develop congestive heart failure and coronary artery disease, and the risk of coronary artery disease appears to be greatest in those with severe long-term AD [110,111].

The association of AD and diabetes mellitus is inconsistent. Recent studies have demonstrated a positive association of AD and DMII [112], while others have found an association with diabetes without specifying type 1 or 2 [113] and/or have not observed an association [108, 114, 115]. It is worth mentioning that the use of topical as well as systemic corticosteroids has been shown to be associated with an increased risk of diabetes and warrants further investigation [115].

The link between AD and obesity in children and adults is less clear. A multicenter case-control study found that children with AD were significantly more likely to have a body mass index (BMI) in the 97th percentile or higher and a waist circumference in the 85th percentile or higher than controls [116]. In addition, AD was found to be associated with a higher percentile of systolic and diastolic blood pressure after adjustment for age, sex, and family history of hypertension [116]. These associations may be influenced by genetics, circulating inflammatory cytokines, lifestyle factors (i.e., smoking, drinking), or shared risk factors such as impaired sleep [1]. Moreover, a systematic review and meta-analysis of 30 observational studies in 2015 reported that being overweight and obese were associated with an increased prevalence of AD in Asian and North American populations [117]. A 2018 systematic review concluded that most of the evidence, especially recent prospective studies, indicated that obesity is positively associated with AD, but this was not uniformly observed in previous cross-sectional studies [118]. This inconsistency may be explained by the difference in study design, the diagnostic criteria of AD, regional variation, and the diverse definitions of overweight/obesity employed in the studies. Conversely, a Canadian cross-sectional survey found AD to be associated with a mild reduction in the risk of hypertension, DMII and stroke after adjusting for age, sex, ethnic background, BMI, smoking status, alcohol intake, sleep, and physical activity [119]. However, the mechanisms underlying these associations are largely unknown. Large prospective cohort studies are required to confirm the association between AD and these cardiometabolic comorbidities.

In summary, the currently available information to date indicates that while adults with AD in some populations have an increased frequency of CV risk factors, such as obesity and hypertension, it is yet unconvincing to conclude that AD represents an independent or clinically significant risk factor for developing cardiometabolic diseases. However, in adults with severe AD, screening for CV diseases and other risk factors for CV diseases may be justified.

2.5. Autoimmune Diseases

Emerging evidence suggests a convincing relationship between autoimmunity and AD [120]. The demonstration that patients with AD usually exhibit IgE autoreactivity to a variety of human protein antigens provokes the probable autoimmune mechanism behind AD pathogenesis [121, 122]. Whether the presence of serum autoreactive IgE, predisposed genetic aberration and/or environmental factors elicit autoreactivity in AD is still controversial. Since some fungal and animal antigens share sequence homologies with human antigens, the fact that human IgE recognizes both exogenous and endogenous human antigens supports the assumption of autoimmunity in AD pathogenesis [120]. It is conceivable that autoreactivity develops in early childhood, especially between 2 and 6 years old, which represents the critical period for IgE autosensitization

[123]. Skin barrier dysfunction, filaggrin gene mutation and perpetual inflammation caused by *S. aureus* colonization have been postulated to contribute to the development of aberrant IgE production in AD. Moreover, constant scratching of itchy AD skin may further deteriorate cutaneous injury, leading to the release of intracellular autoantigens and the development of autoimmune mechanisms [124]. In fact, evidence of autoreactivity is seen in up to 91% of patients with AD, regardless of age, sex, or disease duration [124]. Increasing data continually reported the coexistence of AD with autoimmune diseases, including Crohn's disease, ulcerative colitis, celiac disease, and alopecia areata [113, 114, 125-129]. Conversely, alopecia areata also increases the risk of AD, particularly in those with early-onset and/or having severe forms of alopecia areata (i.e., alopecia totalis and alopecia universalis) [129-132]. Genetic linkage appears to share some roles, as evidenced by the substantial overlapping susceptibility loci in AD and other autoimmune diseases, including alopecia areata and inflammatory bowel disease [133, 134].

2.6. Malignancy

There has been substantial heterogeneity between studies examining the association between AD and various types of cancers. While some evidence proposes lower rates of malignancy among people with allergic diseases, including AD, the risk literally depends on the types of allergic disease, types of cancer and cancer sites [1]. Multiple population-based case-control and cohort studies suggested AD as a protective factor against overall cancers [135-138]. This is partly due to the increased immune surveillance and higher expression of thymic stromal lymphopoietin/Th2 inflammatory markers in people with allergic diseases, leading to inhibition of various types of cancers, including breast cancer, gastric cancer, pancreatic cancer, and melanoma [138, 139]. On the other hand, contradictory evidence suggests that chronic Th2 inflammation associated with AD could also trigger some types of malignancy [140, 141].

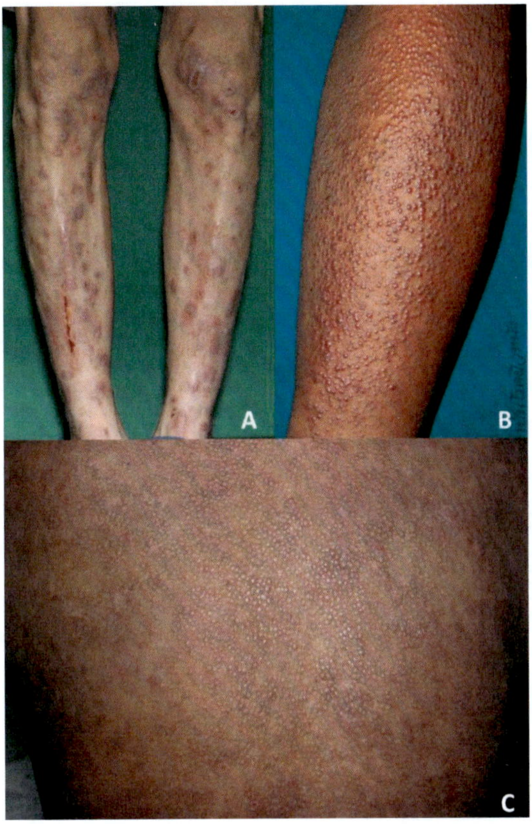

Figure 3. Cutaneous T cell lymphoma: (A) Cutaneous T cell lymphoma can sometimes show overlapping features with atopic dermatitis and may be initially misdiagnosed as severe atopic dermatitis. (B) and (C) Folliculotropic mycosis fungoides, the most common form of cutaneous T cell lymphoma, can present with various skin lesions such as follicle-based patches and plaques which are usually associated with significant pruritus and can be confused with atopic dermatitis.

Although AD has been shown to be associated with lymphoma, the evidence of their relationship remains controversial [137, 142]. A systematic review and meta-analysis in 2015 found a slight increase in lymphoma risk in patients with AD compared with the general population [143]. In addition, the risk of developing cutaneous T cell lymphoma increased with AD severity [144-146]. However, this result must be interpreted with caution because many cutaneous T cell lymphoma cases might have been misdiagnosed and treated as severe AD in the first place

(Figure 3). It is worth mentioning that the relative risk of lymphoma was significantly increased with AD in cohort studies but not in case-control studies [143]. However, due to the considerable discrepancy in study design and diagnostic criteria of case-control studies, a definite conclusion could not be reached. Evidence for the risk of other cutaneous malignancies, such as melanoma and nonmelanoma skin cancer, associated with AD is conflicting. High-quality systematic reviews and meta-analyses have been hampered by the methodological variation among different studies. The reduced daily sunlight exposure due to heat- and sweat-induced pruritus might explain the reduced skin cancer risk in AD [147, 148].

A large systematic review and meta-analysis in 2019, including 8 population-based cohort studies and 48 case-control studies demonstrated a significant association between AD and keratinocyte carcinoma, kidney cancer, lung and respiratory system cancers [149]. Moreover, a recent Taiwanese nationwide cohort study reported a convincing relationship between AD and colorectal carcinoma in both men and women in all age groups, although previous studies have not produced consistent findings [150]. In summary, further studies are essential to confirm these results and to explore the mechanisms underlying a possible association between AD and cancer risk.

2.7. Skin Diseases

Previous studies indicated that up to 37% of patients with AD have clinical evidence of ichthyosis vulgaris [151, 152]. Mutations in the *FLG* gene underlie the pathogenesis of both ichthyosis vulgaris and AD. Furthermore, the clinical severity of ichthyosis vulgaris also positively correlates with AD severity, and the presence of ichthyosis vulgaris may be used to predict an earlier onset disease and a more severe AD phenotype [151]. Hyperlinear palms and keratosis pilaris are the two commonly encountered clinical manifestations in patients with AD and ichthyosis vulgaris. Clinical pictures of ichthyosis vulgaris are showed in Figure 4.

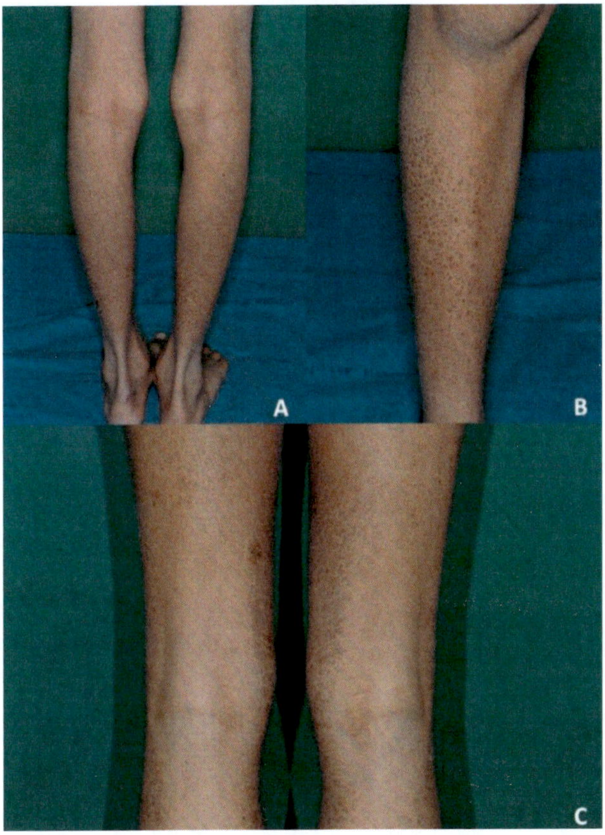

Figure 4. Ichthyosis vulgaris: Ichthyosis vulgaris presents with diffuse, scaly skin with centrally-attached white or light-grey-scales on the trunk and extremities.

Although the literature is conflicting, allergic contact dermatitis (ACD) appears to be a common clinical problem in children and adults with AD [12] (Figure 5). Recent work reported that approximately one-third of children with AD were patch-tested positive with at least one contact allergen [153]. The impaired skin barrier, which allows higher allergen penetration, dysregulated immunity and the frequent application of emollients and various topical medicaments, is assumed to predispose individuals with AD to develop ACD [12]. Common allergens include lanolin, neomycin, formaldehyde, sesquiterpine lactone mix, compositae mix, and fragrance mix, which are common ingredients in AD patients' personal care products [12]. However, a systematic review and meta-analysis in 2017 found no evident difference in contact sensitization between patients with AD and controls [154], while another review presented a lower prevalence of contact allergy among children with AD [153]. Due to the divergence in study designs, patch test methodology, patient characteristics, and criteria for AD, it is difficult to draw any conclusions regarding whether there is a causal relationship between AD and ACD [153]. Although this remains controversial, ACD continues to be an important comorbidity and potential aggravator of AD. Physicians should consider patch testing in patients with AD when clinical ACD is suspected.

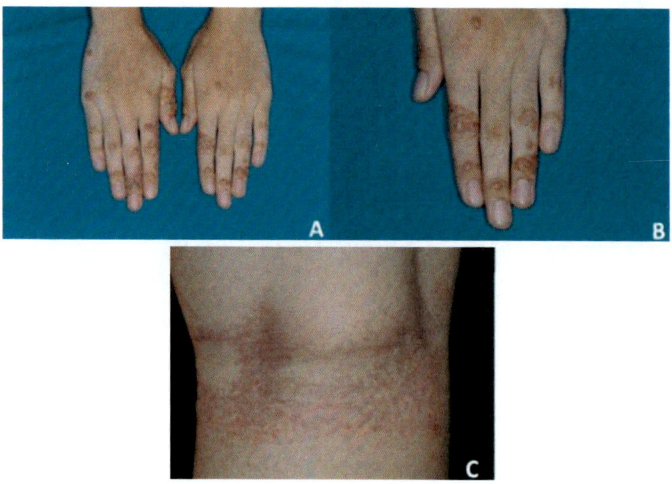

Figure 5. Nickel allergy: (A) and (B) Nickel allergy is one of the most common causes of allergic contact dermatitis. The lesions tend to be intensely itchy and may become red and blistered in acute stage or dry, lichenified and hyperpigmented in chronic stage. (C) The skin of a patient who developed allergic contact dermatitis to skin adhesives showed excoriated erythematous papules coalescing into plaques on the popliteal fossa.

2.8. Eye Diseases

Although ocular involvement only presents in 20-43% of patients with AD, atopic keratoconjunctivitis (AKC) is almost always associated with AD [155]. AKC, a chronic inflammatory ocular condition that can affect patients with AD in any disease course and independent of clinical cutaneous severity, is a severe ocular complication of AD that can result in permanent vision loss if not treated promptly. Complications of AKC include cataracts, keratoconus, infectious keratitis, blepharitis, tear dysfunction, and steroid-induced glaucoma [155]. Apart from AKC, other ocular comorbidities associated with AD could be periocular skin irritation, corneal ulcers, secondary infections, corneal perforation, and retinal detachment [156]. These findings suggest a need for dermatologists to proactively manage their patients with AD with a multidisciplinary approach. When there is moderate to severe ocular irritation, increased erythema, abnormal discharge, or any visual symptoms, immediate referral to an ophthalmologist is indicated.

2.9. Anemia

An increasing prevalence of anemia has been observed in patients with AD as well as other atopic diseases, such as allergic rhinitis and asthma [157], and this association has been reproducible in multiple studies. A Korean cross-sectional investigation found a higher prevalence of iron deficiency anemia and anemia of inflammation in patients with AD when compared with controls, and the difference was significant even after adjustment for demographic characteristics and other risk factors [155]. This finding correlated with previous studies that stated that there was a valid association between AD and anemia in children [158, 159]. A United States cross-sectional survey of caregiver-reported and self-reported data on children and adolescents with atopic disorders, including AD, asthma, hay fever and food allergy, found an increased risk of anemia, especially microcytic anemia [158]. In addition, another Korean cross-sectional study reported an association between atopic diseases and iron deficiency anemia (IDA) after adjusting for confounders, and the risk for IDA was more pronounced in those with multiple atopic comorbidities [159]. Since AD is associated with some chronic inflammatory medical conditions, such as autoimmune and neuropsychiatric diseases, some authors postulated that

IDA or anemia of chronic disease might be related to the inflammatory state of atopic conditions [159]. However, to better understand the etiology of anemia in atopic diseases and elucidate the mechanism behind these links, further study is indispensable.

Conclusion

AD has an enormous impact on patients' quality of life. Aside from cutaneous signs and symptoms, recent data have demonstrated a complex relationship between AD and other allergic and nonallergic comorbidities. Common allergic comorbidities of AD include asthma, food allergy, allergic rhinitis, and eosinophilic esophagitis. Furthermore, AD is related to nonallergic conditions such as psychosocial disorders, autoimmune diseases, anemia, and cutaneous and extracutaneous infections of bacterial, viral, and fungal origins. Whether AD is associated with an increased risk of CV diseases, obesity, hypertension, metabolic syndrome, and malignancy is still controversial, and the mechanisms of their correlation remain unclear. Caring physicians should be aware of potential comorbidities of AD and combine them into clinical decision making, as screening and early detection can improve longevity and overall quality of life in patients with AD.

Conflict of Interest

The authors declare no conflicts of interest.

Acknowledgments

The authors wish to thank Kamonwat Chongkoltanalab (Bangkok, Thailand) for graphic illustration and Michiyo Matsumoto for secretarial assistance. This project was funded by a Grant-in-Aid for Scientific Research from the Ministry of Education, Culture, Sports, Science and Technology, Japan (Grant Number: 26461703 to F.N.).

REFERENCES

[1] Paller, A., Jaworski, J.C., Simpson, E.L., Boguniewicz, M., Russell, J.J., Block, J.K., Tofte, S., Dunn, J.D., Feldman, S.R., Clark, A.R., Schwartz, G. and Eichenfield, L.F. (2018). Major comorbidities of atopic dermatitis: beyond allergic disorders. *Am J Clin Dermatol*, 19(6): 821-38. doi: 10.1007/s40257-018-0383-4.

[2] Thyssen, J.P., McFadden, J.P. and Kimber, I. (2014). The multiple factors affecting the association between atopic dermatitis and contact sensitization. *Allergy*, 69(1): 28-36. doi: 10.1111/all.12358.

[3] Ruff, S.M.D., Engebretsen, K.A., Zachariae, C., Johansen, J.D., Silverberg, J.I., Egeberg, A. and Thyssen, J.P. (2018). The association between atopic dermatitis and hand eczema: a systematic review and meta-analysis. *Br J Dermatol*, 178(4): 879-88. doi: 10.1111/bjd.16147.

[4] Leonard, A. and Guttman-Yassky, E. (2019). The unique molecular signatures of contact dermatitis and implications for treatment. *Clin Rev Allergy Immunol*, 56(1): 1-8. doi: 10.1007/s12016-018-8685-0.

[5] Brunner, P.M., Silverberg, J.I., Guttman-Yassky, E., Paller, A.S., Kabashima, K., Amagai, M., Luger, T.A., Deleuran, M., Werfel, T., Eyerich, K., Stingl, G. and councilors of the international eczema council. (2017). Increasing comorbidities suggest that atopic dermatitis is a systemic disorder. *J Invest Dermatol*, 137(1): 18-25. doi:10.1016/j.jid.2016.08.022.

[6] Silverberg, J.I. (2019). Comorbidities and the impact of atopic dermatitis. *Ann Allergy Asthma Immunol*, 123(2): 144-51. doi: 10.1016/j.anai.2019.04.020.

[7] Spergel, J.M. (2010). From atopic dermatitis to asthma: the atopic march. *Ann Allergy Asthma Immunol*, 105(2): 99-106. doi: 10.1016/j.anai.2009.10.002.

[8] Von Kobyletzki, L.B., Bornehag, C.G., Hasselgren, M., Larsson, M., Lindström, C.B. and Svensson, Å. (2012). Eczema in early childhood is strongly associated with the development of asthma and rhinitis in a prospective cohort. *BMC Dermatol*, 12: 11. doi: 10.1186/1471-5945-12-11.

[9] Bantz, S.K., Zhu, Z. and Zheng, T. (2014). The atopic march: progression from atopic dermatitis to allergic rhinitis and asthma. *J Clin Cell Immunol*, 5(2): 202. doi: 10.4172/2155-9899.1000202.

[10] Wan, J., Mitra, N., Hoffstad, O.J., Gelfand, J.M., Yan, A.C. and Margolis, D.J. (2017). Variations in risk of asthma and seasonal allergies between early- and late-onset pediatric atopic dermatitis: a cohort study. *J Am Acad Dermatol*, 77(4): 634-640. doi: 10.1016/j.jaad.2017.06.013.

[11] Thyssen, J.P., Johansen, J.D., Linneberg, A. and Menne, T. (2010). The epidemiology of hand eczema in the general population–prevalence and main findings. *Contact Dermatitis*, 62(2): 75-87. doi: 10.1111/j.1600-0536.2009.01669.x.

[12] Owen, J.L., Vakharia, P.P. and Silverberg, J.I. (2018). The role and diagnosis of allergic contact dermatitis in patients with atopic dermatitis. *Am J Clin Dermatol*, 19(3): 293-302. doi: 10.1007/s40257-017-0340-7.

[13] Eigenmann, P.A. and Calza, A.M. (2000). Diagnosis of IgE-mediated food allergy among Swiss children with atopic dermatitis. *Pediatr Allergy Immunol*, 11(2): 95. doi: 10.1034/j.1399-3038.2000.00071.x.

[14] García, C., El-Qutob, D., Martorell, A., Febrer, I., Rodríguez, M., Cerdá, J.C. and Félix, R. (2007). Sensitization in early age to food allergens in children with atopic dermatitis. *Allergol Immunopathol* (Madr), 35(1): 15-20. doi: 10.1157/13099090.

[15] Lowe, A.J., Leung, D.Y.M., Tang, M.L.K., Su, J.C. and Allen, K.J. (2018). The skin as a target for prevention of the atopic march. *Ann*

Allergy Asthma Immunol, 120(2): 145-51. doi: 10.1016/j.anai. 2017.11.023.

[16] Dharmage, S.C., Lowe, A.J., Matheson, M.C., Burgess, J.A., Allen, K.J. and Abramson, M.J. (2014). Atopic dermatitis and the atopic march revisited. *Allergy*, 69(1): 17-27. doi: 10.1111/all.12268.

[17] Bartnikas, L.M., Gurish, M.F., Burton, O.T., Leisten, S., Janssen, E., Oettgen, H.C., Beaupré, J., Lewis, C.N., Austen, K.F., Schulte, S., Hornick, J.L., Geha, R.S. and Oyoshi, M.K. (2013). Epicutaneous sensitization results in IgE-dependent intestinal mast cell expansion and food-induced anaphylaxis. *J Allergy Clin Immunol*, 131(2): 451-60.e1-6. doi: 10.1016/j.jaci.2012.11.032.

[18] Brough, H.A., Liu, A.H., Sicherer, S., Makinson, K., Douiri, A., Brown, S.J., Stephens, A.C., Irwin McLean, W.H., Turcanu, V., Wood, R.A., Jones, S.M., Burks, W., Dawson, P., Stablein, D., Sampson, H. and Lack, G. (2015). Atopic dermatitis increases the effect of exposure to peanut antigen in dust on peanut sensitization and likely pea nut allergy. *J Allergy Clin Immunol*, 135(1): 164-70. doi:10.1016/j.jaci.2014.10.007.

[19] Leung, D.Y. and Guttman-Yassky, E. (2014). Deciphering the complexities of atopic dermatitis: shifting paradigms in treatment approaches. *J Allergy Clin Immunol*, 134(4): 769-79. doi: 10.1016/j. jaci.2014.08.008.

[20] Irvine, A.D., McLean, W.H. and Leung, D.Y. (2011). Filaggrin mutations associated with skin and allergic diseases. *N Engl J Med*, 365(14): 1315-27. doi: 10.1056/NEJMra1011040.

[21] Rodríguez, E., Baurecht, H., Herberich, E., Wagenpfeil, S., Brown, S.J., Cordell, H.J., Irvine, A.D. and Weidinger, S. (2009). Meta-analysis of filaggrin polymorphisms in eczema and asthma: robust risk factors in atopic disease. *J Allergy Clin Immunol*, 123(6): 1361-70.e7. doi: 10.1016/j.jaci.2009.03.036.

[22] Van den Oord, R.A. and Sheikh, A. (2009). Filaggrin gene defects and risk of developing allergic sensitization and allergic disorders: systematic review and meta-analysis. *BMJ*, 339: b2433. doi: 10.1136/bmj.b2433.

[23] Gutowska-Owsiak, D., Schaupp, A.L., Salimi, M., Taylor, S. and Ogg, G.S. (2011). Interleukin-22 downregulates filaggrin expression and affects expression of profilaggrin processing enzymes. *Br J Dermatol*, 165(3): 492-8. doi: 10.1111/j.1365-2133.2011.10400.x.

[24] Howell, M.D., Kim, B.E., Gao, P., Grant, A.V., Boguniewicz, M., Debenedetto, A., Schneider, L., Beck, L.A., Barnes, K.C. and Leung, D.Y. (2007). Cytokine modulation of atopic dermatitis filaggrin skin expression. *J Allergy Clin Immunol*, 120(1): 150-5. doi: 10.1016/j.jaci.2007.04.031.

[25] Hvid, M., Vestergaard, C., Kemp, K., Christensen, G.B., Deleuran, B. and Deleuran, M. (2011). IL-25 in atopic dermatitis: a possible link between inflammation and skin barrier dysfunction? *J Invest Dermatol*, 131(1): 150-7. doi: 10.1038/jid.2010.277.

[26] Pellerin, L., Henry, J., Hsu, C.Y., Balica, S., Jean-Decoster, C., Méchin, M.C., Hansmann, B., Rodriguez, E., Weindinger, S., Schmitt, A.M., Serre, G., Paul, C. and Simon, M. (2013). Defects of filaggrin-like proteins in both lesional and nonlesional atopic skin. *J Allergy Clin Immunol*, 131(4): 1094-102. doi: 10.1016/j.jaci.2012.12.1566.

[27] Chalmers, J.R., Haines, R.H., Mitchell, E.J., Thomas, K.S., Brown, S.J., Ridd, M., Lawton, S., Simpson, E.L., Cork, M.J., Sach, T.H., Bradshaw, L.E., Montgomery, A.A., Boyle, R.J. and Williams, H.C. (2017). Effectiveness and cost-effectiveness of daily all-over-body application of emollient during the first year of life for preventing atopic eczema in high-risk children (The BEEP trial): protocol for a randomized controlled trial. *Trials*, 18(1): 343. doi: 10.1186/s13063-017-2031-3.

[28] Simpson, E.L., Chalmers, J.R., Hanifin, J.M., Thomas, K.S., Cork, M.J., McLean, W.H., Brown, S.J., Chen, Z., Chen, Y. and Williams, H.C. (2014). Emollient enhancement of the skin barrier from birth offers effective atopic dermatitis prevention. *J Allergy Clin Immunol*, 134(4): 818-23. doi: 10.1016/j.jaci.2014.08.005.

[29] Horimukai, K., Morita, K., Narita, M., Kondo, M., Kitazawa, H., Nozaki, M., Shigematsu, Y., Yoshida, K., Niizeki, H., Motomura,

K., Sago, H., Takimoto, T., Inoue, E., Kamemura, N., Kido, H., Hisatsune, J., Sugai, M., Murota, H., Katayama, I., Sasaki, T., Amagai, M., Morita, H., Matsuda, A., Matsumoto, K., Saito, H. and Ohya, Y. (2014). Application of moisturizer to neonates prevents development of atopic dermatitis. *J Allergy Clin Immunol*, 134(4): 824-30. doi: 10.1016/j.jaci.2014.07.060.

[30] Czarnowicki, T., Malajian, D., Khattri, S., Correa da Rosa, J., Riana Dutt, Finney., R., Dhingra., N., Xiangyu, P., Xu, H., Estrada, D.Y., Zheng, X., Gilleaudeau, P., Sullivan-Whalen, M., Mayte Suaréz-Fariñas, M., Shemer, A., Krueger, G.J. and Guttman-Yassky, E. (2016). Petrolatum: barrier repair and antimicrobial responses underlying this "inert" moisturizer. *J Allergy Clin Immunol*, 137: 1091-102. doi: 10.1016/j.jaci.2015.08.013.

[31] Yaghmaie, P., Koudelka, C.W. and Simpson, E.L. (2013). Mental health comorbidity in patients with atopic dermatitis. *J Allergy Clin Immunol*, 131(2): 428-33. doi: 10.1016/j.jaci.2012.10.041.

[32] Slattery, M.J., Essex, M.J., Paletz, E.M., Vanness, E.R., Infante, M., Rogers, G.M. and Gern, J.E. (2011). Depression, anxiety, and dermatologic quality of life in adolescents with atopic dermatitis. *J Allergy Clin Immunol*, 128(3): 668-71. doi: 10.1016/j.jaci.2011.05.003.

[33] Lewis-Jones, S. (2006). Quality of life and childhood atopic dermatitis: the misery of living with childhood eczema. *Int J Clin Pract*, 60(8): 984-92. doi: 10.1111/j.1742-1241.2006.01047.x.

[34] Kage, P., Simon, J.C. and Treudler, R. (2020). Atopic dermatitis and psychosocial comorbidities. *J Dtsch Dermatol Ges,* 18(2): 93-102. doi: 10.1111/ddg.14029.

[35] Yu, S.H. and Silverberg, J.I. (2015). Association between atopic dermatitis and depression in US adults. *J Invest Dermatol*, 135(12): 3183–6. doi: 10.1038/jid.2015.337.

[36] Kim, S.H., Hur, J., Jang, J.Y., Park, H.S., Hong, C.H., Son, S.J. and Chang, K.J. (2015). Psychological distress in young adult males with atopic dermatitis: a cross-sectional study. *Medicine (Baltimore),* 94(23): e949. doi: 10.1097/MD.0000000000000949.

[37] Dieris-Hirche, J., Gieler, U., Petrak, F., Milch, W., Te Wildt, B., Dieris, B. and Herpertz, S. (2017). Suicidal ideation in adult patients with atopic dermatitis: a German cross-sectional study. *Acta Derm Venereol*, 97(10): 1189–95. doi: 10.2340/00015555-2741.

[38] Lee, S. and Shin, A. (2017). Association of atopic dermatitis with depressive symptoms and suicidal behaviors among adolescents in Korea: the 2013 Korean youth risk behavior survey. *BMC Psychiatry*, 17(1): 3. doi: 10.1186/s12888-016-1160-7.

[39] Patel, K.R., Immaneni, S., Singam, V., Rastogi, S. and Silverberg, J.I. (2019). Association between atopic dermatitis, depression, and suicidal ideation: a systematic review and meta-analysis. *J Am Acad Dermatol*, 80(2): 402-10. doi: 10.1016/j.jaad.2018.08.063.

[40] Thyssen, J.P., Hamann, C.R., Linneberg, A., Dantoft, T.M., Skov, L., Gislason, G.H., Wu, J.J. and Egeberg A. (2018). Atopic dermatitis is associated with anxiety, depression, and suicidal ideation, but not with psychiatric hospitalization or suicide. *Allergy*, 73(1): 214-20. doi: 10.1111/all.13231.

[41] Rønnstad, A.T.M., Halling-Overgaard, A.S., Hamann, C.R., Skov, L., Egeberg, A. and Thyssen, J.P. (2018). Association of atopic dermatitis with depression, anxiety, and suicidal ideation in children and adults: a systematic review and meta-analysis. *J Am Acad Dermatol*, 79(3): 448-56. doi: 10.1016/j.jaad.2018.03.017.

[42] Cheng, C.M., Hsu, J.W., Huang, K.L., Bai, Y.M., Su, T.P., Li, C.T., Yang, A.C., Chang, W.H., Chen, T.J., Tsai, S.J. and Chen, M.H. (2015). Risk of developing major depressive disorder and anxiety disorders among adolescents and adults with atopic dermatitis: a nationwide longitudinal study. *J Affect Disord*, 178: 60-5. doi: 10.1016/j.jad.2015.02.025.

[43] Mina, S., Jabeen, M., Singh, S. and Verma, R. (2015). Gender differences in depression and anxiety among atopic dermatitis patients. *Indian J Dermatol*, 60(2): 211. doi: 10.4103/0019-5154.152564.

[44] Brew, B.K., Lundholm, C., Gong, T., Larsson, H. and Almqvist, C. (2018). The familial aggregation of atopic diseases and depression or

anxiety in children. *Clin Exp Allergy*, 48(6): 703-11. doi: 10.1111/cea.13127.

[45] Raison, C.L., Capuron, L. and Miller, A.H. (2006). Cytokines sing the blues: inflammation and the pathogenesis of depression. *Trends Immunol*, 27(1): 24-31. doi: 10.1016/j.it.2005.11.006.

[46] Wachholz, S., Knorr, A., Mengert, L., Plümper, J., Sommer, R., Juckel, G. and Friebe, A. (2017). Interleukin-4 is a participant in the regulation of depressive-like behavior. *Behav Brain Res*, 326: 165-72. doi: 10.1016/j.bbr.2017.03.020.

[47] De la O-Escamilla, N.O. and Sidbury, R. (2020). Atopic dermatitis: update on pathogenesis and therapy. *Pediatr Ann*, 49(3): e140-e146. doi: 10.3928/19382359-20200217-01.

[48] Bissonnette, R., Papp, K.A., Poulin, Y., Gooderham, M., Raman, M., Mallbris, L., Wang, C., Purohit, V., Mamolo, C., Papacharalambous, J. and Ports, W.C. (2016). Topical tofacitinib for atopic dermatitis: a phase IIa randomized trial. *Br J Dermatol*, 175(5): 902-11. doi: 10.1111/bjd.14871.

[49] Guttman-Yassky, E., Silverberg, J.I., Nemoto, O., Forman, S.B., Wilke, A., Prescilla, R., de la Peña, A., Nunes, F.P., Janes, J., Gamalo, M., Donley, D., Paik, J., DeLozier, A.M., Nickoloff, B.J. and Simpson, E.L. (2019). Baricitinib in adult patients with moderate-to-severe atopic dermatitis: a phase 2 parallel, double-blinded, randomized placebo-controlled multiple-dose study. *J Am Acad Dermatol*, 80(4): 913-21. doi: 10.1016/j.jaad.2018.01.018.

[50] Simpson, E.L., Bieber, T., Guttman-Yassky, E., Beck, L.A., Blauvelt, A., Cork, M.J., Silverberg, J.I., Deleuran, M., Kataoka, Y., Lacour, J.P., Kingo, K., Worm, M., Poulin, Y., Wollenberg, A., Soo, Y., Graham, N.M., Pirozzi, G., Akinlade, B., Staudinger, H., Mastey, V., Eckert, L., Gadkari, A., Stahl, N., Yancopoulos, G.D., Ardeleanu, M. and SOLO 1 and SOLO 2 Investigators. (2016). Two phase 3 trials of dupilumab versus placebo in atopic dermatitis. *N Engl J Med*, 375: 2335-48. doi: 10.1056/NEJMoa1610020.

[51] Yaghmaie, P., Koudelka, C.W. and Simpson, E.L. (2013). Mental health comorbidity in patients with atopic dermatitis. *J Allergy Clin Immunol*, 131(2): 428-33. doi: 10.1016/j.jaci.2012.10.041.

[52] Chen, M.H., Su, T.P., Chen, Y.S., Hsu, J.W., Huang, K.L., Chang, W.H., Chen, T.J., Pan, T.L. and Bai, Y.M. (2014). Is atopy in early childhood a risk factor for ADHD and ASD? A longitudinal study. *J Psychosom Res*, 77(4): 316-21. doi: 10.1016/j.jpsychores. 2014.06.006.

[53] Shyu, C.S., Lin, H.K., Lin, C.H. and Fu, L.S. (2012). Prevalence of attention-deficit/hyperactivity disorder in patients with pediatric allergic disorders: a nationwide, population-based study. *J Microbiol Immunol Infect*, 45(3): 237-42. doi: 10.1016/j.jmii.2011.11.008.

[54] Schmitt, J., Buske-Kirschbaum, A. and Roessner, V. (2010). Is atopic disease a risk factor for attention-deficit/hyperactivity disorder? A systematic review. *Allergy*, 65(12): 1506-24. doi: 10.1111/j.1398-9995.2010.02449.x.

[55] Strom, M.A., Fishbein, A.B., Paller, A.S. and Silverberg, J.I. (2016). Association between atopic dermatitis and attention deficit hyperactivity disorder in U.S. children and adults. *Br J Dermatol,* 175(5): 920-9. doi: 10.1111/bjd.14697.

[56] Tsai, J.D., Chang, S.N., Mou, C.H., Sung, F.C. and Lue, K.H. (2013). Association between atopic diseases and attention-deficit/hyperactivity disorder in childhood: a population-based case-control study. *Ann Epidemiol*, 23(4): 185-8. doi: 10.1016/j. annepidem.2012.12.015.

[57] Schmitt, J., Apfelbacher, C., Heinrich, J., Weidinger, S. and Romanos, M. (2013). Association of atopic eczema and attention-deficit/hyperactivity disorder – meta-analysis of epidemiologic studies. *Z Kinder Jugendpsychiatr Psychother*, 41(1): 35-42. doi: 10.1024/1422-4917/a000208.

[58] Schmitt, J., Buske-Kirschbaum, A., Tesch, F., Trikojat, K., Stephan, V., Abraham, S., Bauer, A., Nemat, K., Plessow, F. and Roessner, V. (2018). Increased attention-deficit/hyperactivity symptoms in atopic

dermatitis are associated with history of antihistamine use. *Allergy*, 73(3): 615-26. doi: 10.1111/all.13326.

[59] Billeci, L., Tonacci, A., Tartarisco, G., Ruta, L., Pioggia, G. and Gangemi, S. (2015). Association between atopic dermatitis and autism spectrum disorders: a systematic review. *Am J Clin Dermatol*, 16(5): 371-88. doi: 10.1007/s40257-015-0145-5.

[60] Schmitt, J., Apfelbacher, C., Chen, C.M., Romanos, M., Sausenthaler, S., Koletzko, S., Bauer, C.P., Hoffmann, U., Krämer, U., Berdel, D., von Berg, A., Wichmann, H.E. and Heinrich, J; German Infant Nutrition Intervention plus Study Group. (2010). Infant-onset eczema in relation to mental health problems at age 10 years: results from a prospective birth cohort study (German infant nutrition intervention plus). *J Allergy Clin Immunol*, 125(2): 404-10. doi: 10.1016/j.jaci.2009.10.055.

[61] Strom, M.A., Fishbein, A.B., Paller, A.S. and Silverberg, J.I. (2016). Association between atopic dermatitis and attention deficit hyperactivity disorder in U.S. children and adults. *Br J Dermatol*, 175(5): 920-9. doi: 10.1111/bjd.14697.

[62] Romanos, M., Gerlach, M., Warnke, A. and Schmitt, J. (2010). Association of attention-deficit/hyperactivity disorder and atopic eczema modified by sleep disturbance in a large population-based sample. *J Epidemiol Community Health*, 64(3): 269-73. doi: 10.1136/jech.2009.093534.

[63] Buske-Kirschbaum, A., Schmitt, J., Plessow, F., Romanos, M., Weidinger, S. and Roessner, V. (2013). Psychoendocrine and psychoneuroimmunological mechanisms in the comorbidity of atopic eczema and attention deficit/hyperactivity disorder. *Psychoneuro-endocrinology*, 38(1): 12-23. doi: 10.1016/j.psyneuen.2012.09.017.

[64] Pedersen, M.S., Benros, M.E., Agerbo, E., Børglum, D.A. and Mortensen, P.B. (2012). Schizophrenia in patients with atopic disorders with particular emphasis on asthma: a Danish population-based study. *Schizophr Res*, 138(1): 58-62. doi: 10.1016/j.schres.2012.02.019.

[65] Okusaga, O., Hamilton, R.G., Can, A., Igbide, A., Giegling, I., Hartmann, A.M., Konte, B., Friedl, M., Reeves, G.M., Rujescu, D. and Postolache, T.T. (2014). Phadiatop seropositivity in schizophrenia patients and controls: a preliminary study. *AIMS public Heal*, 1(2): 43-50. doi: 10.3934/publichealth.2014.2.43.

[66] Garg, N. and Silverberg, J.I. (2014). Association between childhood allergic disease, psychological comorbidity, and injury requiring medical attention. *Ann Allergy Asthma Immunol*, 112(6): 525-32. doi: 10.1016/j.anai.2014.03.006.

[67] Gupta, M.A., Vujcic, B. and Gupta, A.K. (2017). Dissociation and conversion symptoms in dermatology. *Clin Dermatol*, 35(3): 267-72. doi: 10.1016/j.clindermatol.2017.01.003.

[68] Leyden, J.J., Marples, R.R. and Kligman, A.M. (1974). *Staphylococcus aureus* in the lesions of atopic dermatitis. *Br J Dermatol*. 90(5): 525-30.

[69] Smits, J.P.H., Ederveen, THA., Rikken, G., van den Brink, N.J.M., van Vlijmen-Willems, I.M.J.J., Boekhorst, J., Kamsteeg, M., Schalkwijk, J., van Hijum, S.A.F.T., Zeeuwen, P.L.J.M. and van den Bogaard, E.H. (2020). Targeting the cutaneous microbiota in atopic dermatitis by coal tar via AHR-dependent induction of antimicrobial peptides. *J Invest Dermatol*, 140(2): 415-24.e10. doi: 10.1016/j.jid.2019.06.142.

[70] Kong, H.H., Oh, J., Deming, C., Conlan, S., Grice, E.A., Beatson, M.A., Nomicos, E., Polley, E.C., Komarow, H.D.; NISC Comparative Sequence Program, Murray, P.R., Turner, M.L. and Segre, J.A. (2012). Temporal shifts in the skin microbiome associated with disease flares and treatment in children with atopic dermatitis. *Genome Res*, 22(5): 850-9. doi: 10.1101/gr.131029.111.

[71] Narla, S. and Silverberg, J.I. (2018). Association between atopic dermatitis and serious cutaneous, multiorgan and systemic infections in US adults. *Ann Allergy Asthma Immunol*, 120(1): 66-72. doi: 10.1016/j.anai.2017.10.019.

[72] Hayashida, S., Furusho, N., Uchi, H., Miyazaki, S., Eiraku, K., Gondo, C., Tsuji, G., Hachisuka, J., Fukagawa, S., Kido, M.,

Nakahara, T., Moroi, Y., Hayashi, J., Hagihara, A. and Furue, M. (2010). Are lifetime prevalence of impetigo, molluscum and herpes infection really increased in children having atopic dermatitis? *J Dermatol Sci*, 60(3): 173-8. doi: 10.1016/j.jdermsci.2010.09.003.

[73] Chen, C.F., Wu, K.G., Hsu, M.C. and Tang, R.B. (2001). Prevalence and relationship between allergic diseases and infectious diseases. *J Microbiol Immunol Infect*, 34(1): 57-62.

[74] Hsu, D.Y., Shinkai, K. and Silverberg, J.I. (2018). Epidemiology of eczema herpeticum in hospitalized US children: analysis of a nationwide cohort. *J Invest Dermatol*, 138(2): 265-72. doi: 10.1016/j.jid.2017.08.039.

[75] Mathes, E.F., Oza, V., Frieden, I.J., Cordoro, K.M., Yagi, S., Howard, R., Kristal, L., Ginocchio, C.C., Schaffer, J., Maguiness, S., Bayliss, S., Lara-Corrales, I., Garcia-Romero, M.T., Kelly, D., Salas, M., Oberste, M.S., Nix, W.A., Glaser, C. and Antaya, R. (2013). "Eczema coxsackium" and unusual cutaneous findings in an enterovirus outbreak. *Pediatrics*, 132(1): e149-57. doi: 10.1542/peds.2012-3175.

[76] Strom, M.A. and Silverberg, J.I. (2017). Association between atopic dermatitis and extracutaneous infections in US adults. *Br J Dermatol*, 176(2): 495-7. doi: 10.1111/bjd.14708.

[77] Silverberg, J.I. and Silverberg, N.B. (2014). Childhood atopic dermatitis and warts are associated with increased risk of infection: a US population-based study. *J Allergy Clin Immunol*, 133(4): 1041-7. doi: 10.1016/j.jaci.2013.08.012.

[78] McCollum, A.M., Holman, R.C., Hughes, C.M., Mehal, J.M., Folkema, A.M., Redd, J.T., Cheek, J.E., Damon, I.K. and Reynolds, M.G. (2014). Molluscum contagiosum in a pediatric American Indian population: incidence and risk factors. *PLoS One*, 9(7): e103419. doi: 10.1371/journal.pone.0103419.

[79] Langan, S.M., Abuabara, K., Henrickson, S.E., Hoffstad, O. and Margolis, D.J. (2017). Increased risk of cutaneous and systemic infections in atopic dermatitis: a cohort study. *J Invest Dermatol*, 137(6): 1375-7. doi: 10.1016/j.jid.2017.01.030.

[80] Böhme, M., Lannerö, E., Wickman, M., Nordvall, S.L. and Wahlgren, C.F. (2002). Atopic dermatitis and concomitant disease patterns in children up to 2 years of age. *Acta Derm Venereol*, 82(2): 98-103. doi: 10.1080/000155502529481l2.

[81] Jung, J.A., Kita, H., Yawn, B.P., Boyce, T.G., Yoo, K.H., McGree, M.E., Weaver, A.L., Wollan, P., Jacobson, R.M. and Juhn, Y.J. (2010). Increased risk of serious pneumococcal disease in patients with atopic conditions other than asthma. *J Allergy Clin Immunol*, 125(1): 217-21. doi: 10.1016/j.jaci.2009.10.045.

[82] Silverberg, J.I. and Simpson, E.L. (2013). Association between severe eczema in children and multiple comorbid conditions and increased healthcare utilization. *Pediatr Allergy Immunol*, 24(5): 476-86. doi: 10.1111/pai.12095.

[83] Rotsztejn, H., Frankowska, J., Kamer, B. and Trznadel-Grodzka, E. (2012). Infection cases in infants and small children with atopic dermatitis—own observations. *Postepy Hig Med Dosw* (Online), 66: 96-103.

[84] Fukunaga, N., Okada, Y., Konishi, Y., Murashita, T. and Koyama, T. (2013). Pay attention to valvular disease in the presence of atopic dermatitis. *Circ J*, 77(7): 1862-6. doi: 10.1253/circj.cj-12-1371.

[85] Patel, D. and Jahnke, M.N. (2015). Serious complications from Staphylococcal aureus in atopic dermatitis. *Pediatr Dermatol*, 32(6): 792-6. doi: 10.1111/pde.12665.

[86] Broccardo, C.J., Mahaffey, S., Schwarz, J., Wruck, L., David, G., Schlievert, P.M., Reisdorph, N.A. and Leung, D.Y.M. (2011). Comparative proteomic profiling of patients with atopic dermatitis based on history of eczema herpeticum infection and *Staphylococcus aureus* colonization. *J Allergy Clin Immunol*, 127(1): 186-93. doi: 10.1016/j.jaci.2010.10.033.

[87] De Benedetto, A., Rafaels, N.M., McGirt, L.Y., Ivanov, A.I., Georas, S.N., Cheadle, C., Berger, A.E., Zhang, K., Vidyasagar, S., Yoshida, T., Boguniewicz, M., Hata, T., Schneider, L.C., Hanifin, J.M., Gallo, R.L., Novak, N., Weidinger, S., Beaty, T.H., Leung, D.Y., Barnes, K.C. and Beck, L.A. (2011). Tight junction defects in patients with

atopic dermatitis. *J Allergy Clin Immunol*, 127(3): 773- 86.e1-7. doi: 10.1016/j.jaci.2010.10.018.

[88] Miajlovic, H., Fallon, P.G., Irvine, A.D. and Foster, T.J. (2010). Effect of filaggrin breakdown products on growth of and protein expression by *Staphylococcus aureus*. *J Allergy Clin Immunol*, 126(6): 1184-190.e3. doi: 10.1016/j.jaci.2010.09.015.

[89] Ong, P.Y. and Leung, D.Y. (2010). The infectious aspects of atopic dermatitis. *Immunol Allergy Clin N Am*, 30(3): 309-21. doi: 10.1016/j.iac.2010.05.001.

[90] Grice, K., Sattar, H., Baker, H. and Sharratt, M. (1975). The relationship of transepidermal water loss to skin temperature in psoriasis and eczema. *J Invest Dermatol*, 64(5): 313-5. doi: 10.1111/1523-1747.ep12512258.

[91] Nomura, I., Goleva, E., Howell, M.D., Hamid, Q.A., Ong, P.Y., Hall, C.F., Darst, M.A., Gao, B., Boguniewicz, M., Travers, J.B. and Leung, D.Y. (2003). Cytokine milieu of atopic dermatitis, as compared to psoriasis, skin prevents induction of innate immune response genes. *J Immunol*, 171(6): 3262-9. doi: 10.4049/jimmunol. 171.6.3262.

[92] Guttman-Yassky, E., Nograles, K.E. and Krueger, J.G. (2011). Contrasting pathogenesis of atopic dermatitis and psoriasis. Part I. Clinical and pathologic concepts. *J Allergy Clin Immunol*, 127(5): 1110-8. doi: 10.1016/j.jaci.2011.01.053.

[93] Wilsmann-Theis, D., Hagemann, T., Jordan, J., Bieber, T. and Novak, N. (2008). Facing psoriasis and atopic dermatitis: are there more similarities or more differences? *Eur J Dermatol*, 18(2): 172-80. doi: 10.1684/ejd.2008.0357.

[94] Rieg, S., Steffen, H., Seeber, S., Humeny, A., Kalbacher, H., Dietz, K., Garbe, C. and Schittek, B. (2005). Deficiency of dermcidin-derived antimicrobial peptides in sweat of patients with atopic dermatitis correlates with an impaired innate defense of human skin in vivo. *J Immunol*, 174(12): 8003-10. doi: 10.4049/jimmunol. 174.12.8003.

[95] Kiatsurayanon, C., Ogawa, H. and Niyonsaba, F. (2018). The role of host defense peptide human β-defensins in the maintenance of skin barriers. *Curr Pharm Des*, 24(10): 1092-99. doi: 10.2174/1381612824666180327164445.

[96] Hönzke, S., Wallmeyer, L., Ostrowski, A., Radbruch, M., Mundhenk, L., Schäfer-Korting, M. and Hedtrich, S. (2016). Influence of Th2 cytokines on the cornified envelope, tight junction proteins, and beta-defensins in filaggrin-deficient skin equivalents. *J Invest Dermatol*, 136(3): 631-9. doi: 10.1016/j.jid.2015.11.007.

[97] Cho, S.H., Strickland, I., Tomkinson, A., Fehringer, A.P., Gelfand, E.W. and Leung, D.Y. (2001). Preferential binding of *Staphylococcus aureus* to skin sites of Th2-mediated inflammation in a murine model. *J Invest Dermatol*, 116(5): 658-63. doi: 10.1046/j.0022-202x.2001.01331.x.

[98] Kobayashi, T., Glatz, M., Horiuchi, K., Kawasaki, H., Akiyama, H., Kaplan, D.H., Kong, H.H., Amagai, M. and Nagao, K. (2015). Dysbiosis and *Staphylococcus aureus* colonization drives inflammation in atopic dermatitis. *Immunity*, 42(4): 756-66. doi: 10.1016/j.immuni.2015.03.014.

[99] Volz, T., Skabytska, Y., Guenova, E., Chen, K.M., Frick, J.S., Kirschning, C.J., Kaesler, S., Röcken, M. and Biedermann, T. (2014). Nonpathogenic bacteria alleviating atopic dermatitis inflammation induce IL-10-producing dendritic cells and regulatory Tr1 cells. *J Invest Dermatol*, 134(1): 96-104. doi: 10.1038/jid.2013.291.

[100] Cogen, A.L., Yamasaki, K., Muto, J., Sanchez, K.M., Crotty Alexander, L., Tanios, J., Lai, Y., Kim, J.E., Nizet, V. and Gallo, R.L. (2010). *Staphylococcus epidermidis* antimicrobial delta-toxin (phenol-soluble modulin-gamma) cooperates with host antimicrobial peptides to kill group A *Streptococcus*. *PLoS One*, 5: e8557. doi: 10.1371/journal.pone.0008557.

[101] Lai, Y., Cogen, A.L., Radek, K.A., Park, H.J., Macleod, D.T., Leichtle, A., Ryan, A.F., Di Nardo, A. and Gallo, R.L. (2010). Activation of TLR2 by a small molecule produced by

Staphylococcus epidermidis increases antimicrobial defense against bacterial skin infections. *J Invest Dermatol*, 130(9): 2211-21. doi: 10.1038/jid.2010.123.

[102] Naik, S., Bouladoux, N., Wilhelm, C., Molloy, M.J., Salcedo, R., Kastenmuller, W., Deming, C., Quinones, M., Koo, L., Conlan, S., Spencer, S., Hall, J.A., Dzutsev, A., Kong, H., Campbell, D.J., Trinchieri, G., Segre, J.A. and Belkaid, Y. (2012). Compartmentalized control of skin immunity by resident commensals. *Science*, 337(6098): 1115-9. doi: 10.1126/science. 1225152.

[103] Gueniche, A., Knaudt, B., Schuck, E., Volz, T., Bastien, P., Martin, R., Röcken, M., Breton, L. and Biedermann, T. (2008). Effects of nonpathogenic gram-negative bacterium *Vitreoscilla filiformis* lysate on atopic dermatitis: a prospective, randomized, double-blind, placebo-controlled clinical study. *Br J Dermatol*, 159(6): 1357-63. doi: 10.1111/j.1365-2133.2008.08836.x.

[104] Silverberg, J.I. (2015). Association between childhood atopic dermatitis, malnutrition, and low bone mineral density: a US population-based study. *Pediatr Allergy Immunol*, 26(1): 54-61. doi: 10.1111/pai.12315.

[105] Jolliffe, D.A., Griffiths, C.J. and Martineau, A.R. (2013). Vitamin D in the prevention of acute respiratory infection: systematic review of clinical studies. *J Steroid Biochem Mol Biol*, 136: 321-9. doi: 10.1016/j.jsbmb.2012.11.017.

[106] Ahn, K. (2014). The role of air pollutants in atopic dermatitis. *J Allergy Clin Immunol*, 134(5): 993-9. doi: 10.1016/j.jaci. 2014.09.023.

[107] Ghio, A.J. (2014). Particle exposures and infections. *Infection*, 42(3): 459-67. doi: 10.1007/s15010-014-0592-6.

[108] Thyssen, J.P., Halling-Overgaard, A.S., Andersen, Y.M.F., Gislason, G., Skov, L. and Egeberg, A. (2018). The association with cardiovascular disease and type 2 diabetes in adults with atopic dermatitis: a systematic review and meta-analysis. *Br J Dermatol*, 178(6): 1272-79. doi: 10.1111/bjd.16215.

[109] Silverwood, R.J., Forbes, H.J., Abuabara, K., Ascott, A., Schmidt, M., Schmidt, S.A.J., Smeeth, L. and Langan, S.M. (2018). Severe and predominantly active atopic eczema in adulthood and long term risk of cardiovascular disease: population based cohort study. *BMJ*, 361: k1786. doi: 10.1136/bmj.k1786.

[110] Silverberg, J.I. (2015). Association between adult atopic dermatitis, cardiovascular disease, and increased heart attacks in three population-based studies. *Allergy*, 70(10): 1300-8. doi: 10.1111/all. 12685.

[111] Hjuler, K.F., Bottcher, M., Vestergaard, C., Deleuran, M., Raaby, L., Botker, H.E., Iversen, L. and Kragballe, K. (2015). Increased prevalence of coronary artery disease in severe psoriasis and severe atopic dermatitis. *Am J Med*, 128(12): 1325-34. doi: 10.1016/j.amjmed.2015.05.041.

[112] Thyssen, J.P., Linneberg, A., Carlsen, B.C., Johansen, J.D., Engkilde, K., Hansen, T., Pociot, F., Pedersen, O., Meldgaard, M., Szecsi, P.B., Stender, S. and Menné, T. (2011). A possible association between a dysfunctional skin barrier (filaggrin null-mutation status) and diabetes: a cross-sectional study. *BMJ Open*, 1(1): e000062. doi: 10.1136/bmjopen-2011-000062.

[113] Augustin, M., Radtke, M.A., Glaeske, G., Reich, K., Christophers, E., Schaefer, I. and Jacobi, A. (2015). Epidemiology and comorbidity in children with psoriasis and atopic eczema. *Dermatology*, 231(1): 35-40. doi: 10.1159/000381913.

[114] Radtke, M.A., Schäfer, I., Glaeske, G., Jacobi, A. and Augustin, M. (2017). Prevalence and comorbidities in adults with psoriasis compared to atopic eczema. *J Eur Acad Dermatol Venereol*, 31(1): 151-7. doi: 10.1111/jdv.13813.

[115] Andersen, Y.M.F., Egeberg, A., Gislason, G.H., Skov, L., Knop, F.K. and Thyssen, J.P. (2017). Adult atopic dermatitis and the risk of type 2 diabetes. *J Allergy Clin Immunol*, 139(3): 1057-9. doi: 10.1016/j.jaci.2016.08.049.

[116] Silverberg, J.I., Becker, L., Kwasny, M., Menter, A., Cordoro, K.M. and Paller, A.S. (2015). Central obesity and high blood pressure in

pediatric patients with atopic dermatitis. *JAMA Dermatol*, 151(2): 144-52. doi: 10.1001/jamadermatol.2014.3059.

[117] Zhang, A. and Silverberg, J.I. (2015). Association of atopic dermatitis with being overweight and obese: a systematic review and meta-analysis. *J Am Acad Dermatol*, 72(4): 606-16.e4. doi: 10.1016/j.jaad.2014.12.013.

[118] Ali, Z., Suppli Ulrik, C., Agner, T. and Thomsen, S.F. (2018). Is atopic dermatitis associated with obesity? A systematic review of observational studies. *J Eur Acad Dermatol Venereol*, 32(8): 1246-55. doi: 10.1111/jdv.14879.

[119] Drucker, A.M., Qureshi, A.A., Dummer, T.J.B., Parker, L. and Li, W.Q. (2017). Atopic dermatitis and risk of hypertension, type 2 diabetes, myocardial infarction and stroke in a cross-sectional analysis from the Canadian partnership for tomorrow project. *Br J Dermatol*, 177(4): 1043-51. doi: 10.1111/bjd.15727.

[120] Cipriani, F., Marzatico, A., Ricci, G. (2017). Autoimmune diseases involving skin and intestinal mucosa are more frequent in adolescents and young adults suffering from atopic dermatitis. *J Dermatol*, 44(12): 1341-48. doi: 10.1111/1346-8138.14031.

[121] Mittermann, I., Aichberger, K.J., Bünder, R., Mothes, N., Renz, H. and Valenta, R. (2004). Autoimmunity and atopic dermatitis. *Curr Opin Allergy Clin Immunol*, 4(5): 367–71. doi: 10.1097/00130832-200410000-00007.

[122] Cipriani, F., Ricci, G., Leoni, M.C., Capra, L., Baviera, G., Longo, G., Maiello, N. and Galli, E. (2014). Autoimmunity in atopic dermatitis: biomarker or simply epiphenomenon? *J Dermatol*, 41(7): 569–76. doi: 10.1111/1346-8138.12464.

[123] Navarrete-Dechent, C., Pérez-Mateluna, G., Silva-Valenzuela, S., Vera-Kellet, C. and Borzutzky, A. (2016). Humoral and cellular autoreactivity to epidermal proteins in atopic dermatitis. *Arch Immunol Ther Exp*, 64(6): 435–42. doi: 10.1007/s00005-016-0400-3.

[124] Tang, T.S., Bieber, T. and Williams, H.C. (2012). Does "autoreactivity" play a role in atopic dermatitis? *J Allergy Clin Immunol*, 129(5): 1209-15.e2. doi: 10.1016/j.jaci.2012.02.002.

[125] Andersen, Y.M., Egeberg, A., Gislason, G.H., Skov, L. and Thyssen, J.P. (2017). Autoimmune diseases in adults with atopic dermatitis. *J Am Acad Dermatol*, 76(2): 274-80.e1. doi: 10.1016/j.jaad.2016.08.047.

[126] Kappelman, M.D., Galanko, J.A., Porter, C.Q. and Sandler, R.S. (2011). Association of pediatric inflammatory bowel disease with other immune-mediated diseases. *Arch Dis Child*, 96(11): 1042-6. doi: 10.1136/archdischild-2011-300633.

[127] Schmitt, J., Schwarz, K., Baurecht, H., Hotze, M., Fölster-Holst, R., Rodríguez, E., Lee, Y.A.E., Franke, A., Degenhardt, F. and Lieb, W. (2016). Atopic dermatitis is associated with an increased risk for rheumatoid arthritis and inflammatory bowel disease, and a decreased risk for type 1 diabetes. *J Allergy Clin Immunol*, 137(1): 130-6. doi: 10.1016/j.jaci.2015.06.029.

[128] Ress, K., Annus, T., Putnik, U., Luts, K., Uibo, R. and Uibo, O. (2014). Celiac disease in children with atopic dermatitis. *Pediatr Dermatol*, 31(4): 483-8. doi: 10.1111/pde.12372.

[129] Mohan, G.C. and Silverberg, J.I. (2015). Association of vitiligo and alopecia areata with atopic dermatitis: a systematic review and meta-analysis. *JAMA Dermatol*, 151(5): 522-8. doi: 10.1001/jamadermatol.2014.3324.

[130] Lee, N.R., Kim, B.K., Yoon, N.Y., Lee, S.Y., Ahn, S.Y. and Lee, W.S. (2014). Differences in comorbidity profiles between early-onset and late-onset alopecia areata patients: a retrospective study of 871 Korean patients. *Ann Dermatol*, 26(6): 722-6. doi: 10.5021/ad.2014.26.6.722.

[131] Cho, H.H., Jo, S.J., Paik, S.H., Jeon, H.C., Kim, K.H., Eun, H.C. and Kwon, O.S. (2012). Clinical characteristics and prognostic factors in early-onset alopecia totalis and alopecia universalis. *J Korean Med Sci*, 27(7): 799-802. doi: 10.3346/jkms.2012.27.7.799.

[132] Chu, S.Y., Chen, Y.J., Tseng, W.C., Lin, M.W., Chen, T.J., Hwang, C.Y., Chen, C.C., Lee, D.D., Chang, Y.T., Wang, W.J. and Liu, H.N. (2011). Comorbidity profiles among patients with alopecia areata:

the importance of onset age, a nationwide population-based study. *J Am Acad Dermatol*, 65(5): 949-56. doi: 10.1016/j.jaad.2010.08.032.

[133] Betz, R.C., Pforr, J., Flaquer, A., Redler, S., Hanneken, S., Eigelshoven, S., Kortüm, A.K., Tüting, T., Lambert, J., De Weert, J., Hillmer, A.M., Schmael, C., Wienker, T.F., Kruse, R., Lutz, G., Blaumeiser, B. and Nöthen, M.M. (2007). Loss-of-function mutations in the filaggrin gene and alopecia areata: strong risk factor for a severe course of disease in patients comorbid for atopic disease. *J Invest Dermatol*, 127(11): 2539-43. doi: 10.1038/sj.jid.5700915.

[134] Paternoster, L., Standl, M., Waage, J., Baurecht, H., Hotze, M., Strachan, D.P., Curtin, J.A., Bønnelykke, K., Tian, C., Takahashi, A., Esparza-Gordillo, J., Alves, A.C., Thyssen, J.P., den Dekker, H.T., Ferreira, M.A., Altmaier, E., Sleiman, P.M., Xiao, F.L., Gonzalez, J.R., Marenholz, I., Kalb, B., Yanes, M.P., Xu, C.J., Carstensen, L., Groen-Blokhuis, M.M., Venturini, C., Pennell, C.E., Barton, S.J., Levin, A.M., Curjuric, I., Bustamante, M., Kreiner-Møller, E., Lockett, G.A., Bacelis, J., Bunyavanich, S., Myers, R.A., Matanovic, A., Kumar, A., Tung, J.Y., Hirota, T., Kubo, M., McArdle, W.L., Henderson, A.J., Kemp, J.P., Zheng, J., Smith, G.D., Rüschendorf, F., Bauerfeind, A., Lee-Kirsch, M.A., Arnold, A., Homuth, G., Schmidt, C.O., Mangold, E., Cichon, S., Keil, T., Rodríguez, E., Peters, A., Franke, A., Lieb, W., Novak, N., Fölster-Holst, R., Horikoshi, M., Pekkanen, J., Sebert, S., Husemoen, L.L., Grarup, N., de Jongste, J.C., Rivadeneira, F., Hofman, A., Jaddoe, V.W., Pasmans, S.G., Elbert, N.J., Uitterlinden, A.G., Marks, G.B., Thompson, P.J., Matheson, M.C., Robertson, C.F.; Australian Asthma Genetics Consortium (AAGC), Ried, J.S., Li, J., Zuo, X.B., Zheng, X.D., Yin, X.Y., Sun, L.D., McAleer, M.A., O'Regan, G.M., Fahy, C.M., Campbell, L.E., Macek, M., Kurek, M., Hu, D., Eng, C., Postma, D.S., Feenstra, B., Geller, F., Hottenga, J.J., Middeldorp, C.M., Hysi, P., Bataille, V., Spector, T., Tiesler, C.M., Thiering, E., Pahukasahasram, B., Yang, J.J., Imboden, M., Huntsman, S., Vilor-Tejedor, N., Relton, C.L., Myhre, R., Nystad, W., Custovic, A., Weiss, S.T., Meyers, D.A., Söderhäll, C., Melén, E., Ober, C., Raby,

B.A., Simpson, A., Jacobsson, B., Holloway, J.W., Bisgaard, H., Sunyer, J., Hensch, N.M.P., Williams, L.K., Godfrey, K.M., Wang, C.A., Boomsma, D.I., Melbye, M., Koppelman, G.H., Jarvis, D., McLean, W.I., Irvine, A.D., Zhang, X.J., Hakonarson, H., Gieger, C., Burchard, E.G., Martin, N.G., Duijts, L., Linneberg, A., Jarvelin, M.R., Noethen, M.M., Lau, S., Hübner, N., Lee, Y.A., Tamari, M., Hinds, D.A., Glass, D., Brown, S.J., Heinrich, J., Evans, D.M. and Weidinger, S. (2015). Multi-ancestry genome-wide association study of 21,000 cases and 95,000 controls identifies new risk loci for atopic dermatitis. *Nat Genet*, 47(12): 1449-56. doi: 10.1038/ng.3424.

[135] Egeberg, A., Andersen, Y.M., Gislason, G.H., Skov, L. and Thyssen, J.P. (2017). Prevalence of comorbidity and associated risk factors in adults with atopic dermatitis. *Allergy*, 72(5): 783-91. doi: 10.1111/all.13085.

[136] Hwang, C.Y., Chen, Y.J., Lin, M.W., Chen, T.J., Chu, S.Y., Chen, C.C., Lee, D.D., Chang, Y.T., Wang, W.J. and Liu, H.N. (2012). Cancer risk in patients with allergic rhinitis, asthma and atopic dermatitis: a nationwide cohort study in Taiwan. *Int J Cancer*, 130(5): 1160-7. doi: 10.1002/ijc.26105.

[137] Arana, A., Wentworth, C.E., Fernández-Vidaurre, C., Schlienger, R.G., Conde, E. and Arellano, F.M. (2010). Incidence of cancer in the general population and in patients with or without atopic dermatitis in the UK. *Br J Dermatol*, 163(5): 1036-43. doi: 10.1111/j.1365-2133.2010.09887.x.

[138] Jo, S., Kim, T.J., Lee, H., Min, Y.W., Min, B.H., Lee, J.H., Son, H.J., Rhee, P.L., Baek, S.Y., Kim, S.W. and Kim, J.J. (2018). Associations between atopic dermatitis and risk of gastric cancer: a nationwide population-based study. *Korean J Gastroenterol*, 71(1): 38-44. doi: 10.4166/kjg.2018.71.1.38.

[139] Zhang, Y. and Zhou, B. (2012). Functions of thymic stromal lymphopoietin in immunity and disease. *Immunol Res*, 52(3): 211-23. doi: 10.1007/s12026-012-8264-z.

[140] Josephs, D.H., Spicer, J.F., Corrigan, C.J., Gould, H.J. and Karagiannis, S.N. (2013). Epidemiological associations of allergy,

IgE and cancer. *Clin Exp Allergy*, 43(10): 1110-23. doi: 10.1111/cea.12178.

[141] Rittmeyer, D. and Lorentz, A. (2012). Relationship between allergy and cancer: an overview. *Int Arch Allergy Immunol*, 159(3): 216-25. doi: 10.1159/000338994.

[142] Vajdic, C.M., Falster, M.O., de Sanjose, S., Martínez-Maza, O., Becker, N., Bracci, P.M., Melbye, M., Smedby, K.E., Engels, E.A., Turner, J., Vineis, P., Costantini, A.S., Holly, E.A., Kane, E., Spinelli, J.J., La Vecchia, C., Zheng, T., Chiu, B.C., Dal Maso, L., Cocco, P., Maynadié, M., Foretova, L., Staines, A., Brennan, P., Davis, S., Severson, R., Cerhan, J.R., Breen, E.C., Birmann, B., Cozen, W. and Grulich, A.E. (2009). Atopic disease and risk of non-Hodgkin lymphoma: an InterLymph pooled analysis. *Cancer Res*, 69(16): 6482-9. doi: 10.1158/0008-5472.CAN-08-4372.

[143] Legendre, L., Barnetche, T., Mazereeuw-Hautier, J., Legendre, L., Barnetche, T., Mazereeuw-Hautier, J., Meyer, N., Murrell, D. and Paul, C. (2015). Risk of lymphoma in patients with atopic dermatitis and the role of topical treatment: a systematic review and meta-analysis. *J Am Acad Dermatol*, 72(6): 992-1002. doi: 10.1016/j.jaad.2015.02.1116.

[144] Arellano, F.M., Wentworth, C.E., Arana, A., Fernández, C. and Paul, C.F. (2007). Risk of lymphoma following exposure to calcineurin inhibitors and topical steroids in patients with atopic dermatitis. *J Invest Dermatol*, 127(4): 808-16. doi: 10.1038/sj.jid.5700622.

[145] Arellano, F.M., Arana, A., Wentworth, C.E., Fernández-Vidaurre, C., Schlienger, R.G. and Conde, E. (2009). Lymphoma among patients with atopic dermatitis and/or treated with topical immunosuppressants in the United Kingdom. *J Allergy Clin Immunol*, 123(5): 1111-6, 116.e1-13. doi: 10.1016/j.jaci.2009.02.028.

[146] Margolis, D., Bilker, W., Hennessy, S., Vittorio, C., Santanna, J. and Strom, B.L. (2001). The risk of malignancy associated with psoriasis. *Arch Dermatol*, 137(6): 778-83.

[147] Gandini, S., Stanganelli, I., Palli, D., De Giorgi, V., Masala, G. and Caini, S. (2016). Atopic dermatitis, naevi count and skin cancer risk: a meta-analysis. *J Dermatol Sci*, 84(2): 137-43. doi: 10.1016/j.jdermsci.2016.07.009.

[148] Kallas, M., Rosdahl, I., Fredriksson, M. and Synnerstad, I. (2006). Frequency and distribution pattern of melanocytic naevi in Estonian children and the influence of atopic dermatitis. *J Eur Acad Dermatol Venereol*, 20(2): 143-8. doi: 10.1111/j.1468-3083.2005.01379.x.

[149] Wang, L., Bierbrier, R., Drucker, A.M. and Chan, A.W. (2019). Noncutaneous and cutaneous cancer risk in patients with atopic dermatitis: a systematic review and meta-analysis. *JAMA Dermatol*, 156(2): 158-71. doi: 10.1001/jamadermatol.2019.3786.

[150] Chou, W.Y., Lai, P.Y., Hu, J.M., Hsu, C.H., Chen, Y.C., Tian, Y.F., You, S.L., Hsiao, C.W., Chou, Y.C. and Sun, C.A. (2020). Association between atopic dermatitis and colorectal cancer risk: a nationwide cohort study. *Medicine (Baltimore)*, 99(1): e18530. doi: 10.1097/MD.0000000000018530.

[151] Bremmer, S.F., Hanifin, J.M. and Simpson, E.L. (2008). Clinical detection of ichthyosis vulgaris in an atopic dermatitis clinic: implications for allergic respiratory disease and prognosis. *J Am Acad Dermatol*, 59(1): 72-8. doi: 10.1016/j.jaad.2008.03.029.

[152] Tay, Y.K., Kong, K.H., Khoo, L., Goh, C.L. and Giam, Y.C. (2002). The prevalence and descriptive epidemiology of atopic dermatitis in Singapore school children. *Br J Dermatol*, 146(1): 101-6. doi: 10.1046/j.1365-2133.2002.04566.x.

[153] Simonsen, A.B., Johansen, J.D., Deleuran, M., Mortz, C.G. and Sommerlund, M. (2017). Contact allergy in children with atopic dermatitis: a systematic review. *Br J Dermatol*, 177(2): 395-405. doi: 10.1111/bjd.15628.

[154] Hamann, C.R., Hamann, D., Egeberg, A., Johansen, J.D., Silverberg, J. and Thyssen, J.P. (2017). Association between atopic dermatitis and contact sensitization: a systematic review and meta-analysis. *J Am Acad Dermatol*, 77(1): 70-8. doi: 10.1016/j.jaad.2017.02.001.

[155] Chen, J.J., Applebaum, D.S., Sun, G.S. and Pflugfelder, S.C. (2014). Atopic keratoconjunctivitis: a review. *J Am Acad Dermatol*, 70(3): 569-75. doi: 10.1016/j.jaad.2013.10.036.

[156] Beck, K.M., Seitzman, G.D., Yang, E.J., Sanchez, I.M. and Liao, W. (2019). Ocular co-morbidities of atopic dermatitis. Part I: associated ocular diseases. *Am J Clin Dermatol*, 20(6): 797-805. doi: 10.1007/s40257-019-00455-5.

[157] Rhew, K., Brown, J.D. and Oh, J.M. (2020). Atopic disease and anemia in Korean patients: cross-sectional study with propensity score analysis. *Int J Environ Res Public Health*, 17(6): 1978. doi: 10.3390/ijerph17061978.

[158] Drury, K.E., Schaeffer, M. and Silverberg, J.I. (2016). Association between atopic disease and anemia in US children. *JAMA Pediatr*, 170(1): 29-34. doi: 10.1001/jamapediatrics.2015.3065.

[159] Rhew, K. and Oh, J.M. (2019). Association between atopic disease and anemia in pediatrics: a cross-sectional study. *BMC Pediatr*, 19(1): 455. doi: 10.1186/s12887-019-1836-5.

Biographical Sketches

Chanisa Kiatsurayanon

Affiliation: Institute of Dermatology, Department of Medical Services, Ministry of Public Health, Bangkok, Thailand, Graduate School of Medicine, Rangsit University, Pathumthani, Thailand

Education:

- *May 2003 – Mar 2009*: Faculty of Medicine, Chulalongkorn University, Bangkok, Thailand: Doctor of Medicine (First Class Honors)

- *May 2010 – Mar 2011*: School of Medicine, Cardiff University, Cardiff, Wales, United Kingdom: Diploma in Practical Dermatology
- *Oct 2011 – Apr 2012*: Graduate School of Medicine, Juntendo University, Tokyo, Japan: Research Student, Department of Dermatology and Allergology
- *Apr 2012 – Aug 2015*: Graduate School of Medicine, Juntendo University, Tokyo, Japan: Ph.D. program, Department of Dermatology and Allergology
- *Sep 2015 – June 2017*: Fellowship program in Clinical Dermatology, Institute of Dermatology, Bangkok, Thailand: Clinical Fellow in Dermatology
- *May 2018 – Oct 2018*: Postdoctoral Research Fellowship in Cutaneous Biology, University of Franche-Comté, Besançon, France

Professional Appointments:

- *2017 – Present*: Staff Dermatologist and Lecturer, Institute of Dermatology, Department of Medical Services, Ministry of Public Health, Bangkok, Thailand
- *2019 – Present:* Lecturer, Graduate School of Medicine, Rangsit university, Pathumthani, Thailand

Honors:

- *His Majesty King Bhumibol Honorary Award (1994 and 1996)*: Awarded to Rachavinit School students who have demonstrated outstanding academic ability.
- *Best Student Award (1998)*: Awarded by Srinakharinwirot Patumwan Demonstration School to students with outstanding academic profile and excellent manners.

- *Universal Cultural Exchange Scholarship (Apr 2001 and Oct 2001)*: Awarded by the Universal Cultural Exchange Organization of Thailand. The scholarship enables recipients to study English overseas as a cultural exchange student for one month.
- *Faculty of Medicine, Chulalongkorn University Scholarship (2009)*: Awarded to students with excellent academic profile by the Faculty of Medicine, Chulalongkorn University. The scholarship allows recipients to participate in academic activities of interests at Juntendo University Hospital, Tokyo, Japan.
- *Monbukagakusho Scholarship (2011)*: Awarded by the Ministry of Education, Culture, Sports, Science, and Technology of Japan. One of the most prestigious scholarships offered by the Japanese government.
- *The International Investigative Dermatology Meeting Travel Fellowship Award (2013)*: Awarded by the International Investigative Dermatology to attend the annually meeting held in Edinburgh, Scotland.
- *Young International Dermatologist Award (2014)*: The Sumitomo Mitsui Trust Bank (SMTB) bestows the Young International Dermatologist Award to the most notable junior researchers in dermatology to enhance their motivation in research and education in Japan.
- *Diploma of Dermatological Scientist (2014)*: By the Japanese Society for Investigative Dermatology to develop and support foreign students who engage in dermatology-related research and have demonstrated outstanding performance in dermatology education in Japan.
- *Albert M. Kligman Travel Fellowship Award (2015)*: To support young investigators traveling to the Society for Investigative Dermatology Annual Meeting held in Atlanta, Georgia.

Publications from the Last 3 Years:

1. Thammahong, A., Kiatsurayanon, C., Edwards, S.W., Rerknimitr, P. and Chiewchengchol, D. (2020). The clinical significance of fungi in atopic dermatitis. *Int J Dermatol*, doi: 10.1111/ijd.14941.
2. Inthanachai, T., Thammahong, A., Edwards, S.W., Virakul, S., Kiatsurayanon, C. and Chiewchengchol, D. (2020). The inhibitory effect of human beta-defensin-3 on *Candida Glabrata* isolated from patients with Candidiasis. *Immunol Invest*, doi: 10.1080/08820139.2020.1755307.
3. Kiatsurayanon, C., Ogawa, H. and Niyonsaba, F. (2018) The role of host defense peptide human β-defensins in the maintenance of skin barriers. *Curr Pharm Des*, 24(10):1092-1099. doi: 10.2174/1381612824666180327164445.
4. Chieosilapatham, P., Niyonsaba, F., Kiatsurayanon, C., Okumura, K., Ikeda, S. and Ogawa, H. (2017) The antimicrobial peptide derived from insulin-like growth factor-binding protein 5, AMP-IBP5, regulates keratinocyte functions through Mas-related gene X receptors. *J Dermatol Sci,* 88(1):117-125. doi: 10.1016/j.jdermsci. 2017.05.008.
5. Kiatsurayanon, C., Rojanamatin, J., Sudtikoonaseth, P., Kampirapap, K., Wichaidit, M. and Niyonsaba, F. (2017) Unilateral linear punctate palmoplantar keratoderma: a case report. *Case Rep Dermatol,* 9(1):86-89. doi: 10.1159/000468920.
6. Niyonsaba, F., Kiatsurayanon, C., Chieosilapatham, P. and Ogawa, H. (2017) Friends or Foes? Host defense (antimicrobial) peptides and proteins in human skin diseases. *Exp Dermatol,* 26(11):989-998. doi: 10.1111/exd.13314.

François Niyonsaba

Affiliation: Atopy (Allergy) Research Center, Juntendo University Graduate School of Medicine, Tokyo, Japan. Faculty of International Liberal Arts, Juntendo University.

Research and Professional Experience: François Niyonsaba received his bachelor's degree in medicine and surgery in 1994 and master's degree in Orthopedics (1998) at China Medical University (Liaoning, China). He then joined the Department of Host Defense and Biochemical Research at Juntendo University Graduate School of Medicine (Tokyo, Japan) and received his PhD in 2003. He was appointed as Instructor (2003), Assistant Professor (2006) and Associate Professor (2007) in the Atopy Research Center at Juntendo University. In 2010, he was assigned as Visiting Associate Professor in the Department of Microbiology and Immunology at the University of British Columbia (Vancouver, Canada). In 2015 and 2017, he was promoted to Senior Associate Professor and Full Professor, respectively, in Global Health Studies, Faculty of International Liberal Arts, Juntendo University.

His research interests include "Roles of antimicrobial agents in the skin immunity" (Graduate School of Medicine) and "Global infections" (Faculty of International Liberal Arts). He has published more than 100 papers, reviews and books, and has 17 patents awarded. Niyonsaba's numerous awards/honors include: Outstanding Scholar Award (USA, 2001); Diploma for Dermatological Scientist (Japan, 2003); Takamitsu Sekine Research Award (Japan, 2003); Excellent Young Researchers Overseas Visit Program from the Japan Society for the Promotion of Science JSPS (Japan, 2009); Naito Foundation Fellowship (Japan, 2010), Award for Excellence from the Eastern Asia Dermatology Congress (Korea, 2014), and Honorary Fellowship of the Asian Academy of Dermatology and Venereology (Vietnam, 2017). He is also a scientific adviser in 4 pharmaceutical (cosmetics) companies.

Publications from the Last 3 Years:

1. Chieosilapatham P, Yue H, Ikeda S, Ogawa H, Niyonsaba F. Involvement of the lipoprotein receptor LRP1 in AMP-IBP5-mediated migration and proliferation of human keratinocytes and fibroblasts. *J Dermatol Sci, 2020* (In press).
2. Umehara Y, Toyama S, Tominaga M, Matsuda H, Takahashi N, Kamata Y, Niyonsaba F, Ogawa H, Takamori K: Robust induction of neural crest cells to derive peripheral sensory neurons from human induced pluripotent stem cells. *Sci Rep. 10(1):*4360, 2020.
3. Niyonsaba F, Song P, Yue H, Sutthammikorn N, Umehara Y, Okumura K, Ogawa H. Antimicrobial peptide derived from insulin-like growth factor-binding protein 5 activates mast cells via Mas-related G protein-coupled receptor X2. *Allergy 75(1):*203-207, 2020.
4. Sekihara K, Saitoh K, Yang H, Kawashima H, Kazuno S, Kikkawa M, Arai H, Miida T, Hayashi N, Niyonsaba F, Sasai K, Tabe Y. Low-dose ionizing radiation exposure represses the cell cycle and protein synthesis pathways in in vitro human primary keratinocytes and U937 cell lines. *PLoS One. 13(10):*e0205581, 2018.
5. Murakami T, Suzuki K, Niyonsaba F, Tada H, Reich J, Tamura H, Nagaoka I. MrgX2-mediated internalization of LL-37 and degranulation of human LAD2 mast cells. *Mol Med Rep. 18(6):* 4951-4959, 2018.
6. Kiatsurayanon C, Ogawa H, Niyonsaba F. The role of host defense peptide human β-defensins in the maintenance of skin barriers. *Curr Pharm Des. 24(10):*1079-1091, 2018.
7. Chieosilapatham P, Ikeda S, Ogawa H, Niyonsaba F. Tissue-specific regulation of innate immune responses by human cathelicidin LL-37. *Curr Pharm Des. 24(10):*1092-1099, 2018.
8. Umehara Y, Kamata Y, Tominaga M, Niyonsaba F, Ogawa H, Takamori K. Antimicrobial peptides human LL-37 and β-defensin-3 modulate the expression of nerve elongation factors in human epidermal keratinocytes. *J Dermatol Sci. 88(3):*365-367, 2017.

9. Chieosilapatham P, Ogawa H, Niyonsaba F. Current insights into the role of human β-defensins in atopic dermatitis. *Clin Exp Immunol. 190(2):*155-166, 2017.
10. Yanashima K, Chieosilapatham P, Yoshimoto E, Okumura K, Ogawa H, Niyonsaba F. Innate defense regulator IDR-1018 activates human mast cells through G protein-, phospholipase C-, MAPK- and NF-κB-sensitive pathways. *Immunol Res. 65(4):*920-931, 2017.
11. Chieosilapatham P, Niyonsaba F, Kiatsurayanon C, Okumura K, Ikeda S, Ogawa H. The antimicrobial peptide derived from insulin-like growth factor-binding protein 5, AMP-IBP5, regulates keratinocyte functions through Mas-related gene X receptors. *J Dermatol Sci. 88(1)*:117-125, 2017.
12. Kiatsurayanon C, Rojanamatin J, Sudtikoonaseth P, Kampirapap K, Wichaidit M, Niyonsaba F. Unilateral linear punctate palmoplantar keratoderma: a case report. *Case Rep Dermatol, 9(1):*86–89, 2017.
13. Niyonsaba F, Kiatsurayanon C, Chieosilapatham P, Ogawa H. Friends or Foes? Host defense (antimicrobial) peptides and proteins in human skin diseases. *Exp Dermatol, 26(11)*:989-998, 2017.

In: Atopic Dermatitis
Editor: Andreas Maur

ISBN: 978-1-53618-520-1

Chapter 3

ATOPIC DERMATITIS - THE NUTRITIONAL BIOCHEMISTS' VIEW

Elaine Wat and Ben Chung Lap Chan*
Institute of Chinese Medicine and State Key Laboratory of Research on Bioactivities and Clinical Applications of Medicinal Plants,
The Chinese University of Hong Kong,
Shatin, N.T., Hong Kong, China

ABSTRACT

Atopic dermatitis (AD) is a chronic and pruritic skin condition which affects 10 – 20% of the population worldwide [1]. It can be characterized by pruritus, erythema, vesiculation, exudation, excoriation, crusting, scaling and sometimes lichenification [2]. AD usually starts during infancy or early childhood, and is the commonest childhood skin disease [3]. The lifetime prevalence of AD is estimated to 15-30% in children, and 2-10% in adults. In the past 3 decades, the incidence of AD has increased by 2- to 3-fold in industrialized countries, and this prevalence

* Corresponding Author's E-mail: benchan99@cuhk.edu.hk.

continues to increase [4-6]. As its causes are still poorly understood, the management of AD always presents a great challenge to all clinicians [7, 8]. Although etiology of AD is unclear, genetic factors play a significant role in contributing its prevalence. Nevertheless, recent increase in AD prevalence suggests complex interaction between environmental factors and susceptibility genes may also result in clinical expression of the disorder. Current therapeutic approaches of AD often focus on symptomatic relief rather than cure, and the long-term treatment objectives for AD are aimed at reducing the clinical manifestations, minimizing relapses, and modifying the disease course. These approaches comprise basic skin care for cutaneous rehydration with liberal use of emollients, intermittent use of anti-inflammatory therapy for acute flares and avoidance of triggering factors. Recent increases in the use of TCM, especially in Asia may provide an alternative treatment option. However, the beneficial effects of TCM on AD have not been consistently demonstrated. This book chapter aims to provide a review of AD, from its diagnosis to its recent advances in the treatment options.

Keywords: atopic dermatitis, pathophysiology, emollients, topical steroids, immunomodulators, Traditional Chinese Medicine

PATHOPHYSIOLOGY AND DIAGNOSIS

In 1936, Engman et al. defined AD as "itch that rashes, not an itching rash." This brief but yet straight forward definition very well define the primary symptom of AD is itchiness [9, 10]. It was only up to 1980, Hanifin and Rajka provided a more thorough summary on the definition and diagnostic criteria for AD, suggesting AD should possess major symptoms including itch, chronic relapsing eczema, genetic predisposition, dry skin, lichenification (in adults), and minor symptoms including 3 or more as follow [10, 11]:

- Dry skin
- Ichthyosis
- Palmar hyperlinearity
- Keratosis pilaris
- Type I allergy and increased serum IgE

- Hand and foot dermatitis
- Cheilitis
- Nipple eczema
- Increased presence of *Staphylococcus aureus* and Herpes
- Simplex
- Perifollicular keratosis
- Pityriasis alba
- Early age of onset
- Recurrent conjunctivitis
- Dennie-Morgan infraorbital fold
- Keratoconus
- Cataract
- Orbital darkening
- Facial pallor/facial erythema
- Anterior neck folds
- Itch when sweating
- Intolerance to wool and lipid solvents
- Perifollicular accentuation
- Food intolerance
- Course influenced by environmental and emotional factors
- White dermographism or delayed blanch

While the etiology of AD is complicated and not completely understood, it is generally believed that the pathophysiology of AD involves the collide of skin barrier dysfunction, dysregulation of cell mediated immune responses, IgE mediated hypersensitivity and environmental factors [12, 13].

Skin Barrier Dysfunction

Epidermis is the uppermost epithelial layer of the skin which serves as the physical and functional barrier in preventing moisture loss of water from the body. Clinically, skin barrier defects are the most significant pathologic findings in AD skin [13-16]. The fact that barrier dysfunction was observed in the uninvolved or recovered skin of AD patients suggested barrier abnormalities are an initiator of AD rather than a consequence [17, 18]. It was believed that this disturbed epidermal barrier would lead to penetration of irritative substances and allergens into the skin. Nevertheless, recent evidence demonstrated that immune dysregulation, including the activation of type 2 immune responses, results in impairment of the epidermal barrier. Genetic mutations in the gene filaggrin, which is expressed in the upper layers of the stratum corneum (SC) may also lead to the development of AD [19-22]. Nevertheless, there is no doubt that the skin barrier plays a critical role in host defense against microbial invasion. Once this physical barrier is breached, it could further provoke rapid, innate immune response within the body to further tackle the microbial invasion and replication.

Immune Dysregulation

Keratinocytes and antigen presenting cells in the skin express a number of innate immune receptor known as pattern recognition receptors such as toll-like receptors (TLRs) NOD-like receptors, C-type lectin receptors, and RIG-IY like receptors, which are intrinsic in the initiation of the immune response and recognition of pathogenic antigens [23, 24]. Activation of these receptors could further promote production of antimicrobial peptides, pro-inflammatory cytokines and chemokines that are necessary for protection against foreign pathogens and to limit the penetration of allergens and microbes [23, 24]. Interestingly, AD patients possess reduced function of TLR and reduced production of antimicrobial peptides needed for controlling bacterial growth and viral replication, further predisposing to microbial colonization and chronic skin inflammation [24]. Clinically unaffected skin in AD demonstrates an increased number of Th2 cells and its cytokines (IL-4, IL-13 and IL-31), as compared with normal non-atopic skin [23]. Recent finding suggested that during the initial acute phase of AD, Th22 cytokines are also involved [25]. IL-31 is responsible for inducing severe pruritus as well as inhibiting epidermal differentiation [26]. While IL-4 is important for the differentiation of Th2 cells, IL-13 is critical in generating a cutaneous Th2 response, independent of IL-4. It may also directly induce the expression of IL-5, causing infiltration of eosinophils in the skin, and induces keratinocytes to produce macrophage-derived chemokine (MDC/CCL22), which further attracts CCR4+ Th2 cells [27, 28]. This formation of the inflammatory cytokine cascade would also induce expression of IFN-γ, causing apoptosis of keratinocytes. IL-10 in contrast, is an anti-inflammatory cytokine which would counterbalance the inflammatory reaction by controlling the dendritic cell-induced T cell reactivity in the skin [24].

Dendritic cells are (DC) also recognized as one of the key cells which took part in the initiation of T cell responses in AD. There are two major subtypes of DC in AD lesions, Langerhans' cells (LC) and inflammatory dendritic epidermal cells (IDEC) which express high levels of FceRI [29]. Both LC and IDEC have been shown to be capable of inducing Th2 and Th1 polarization. While LC induce Th1 cells to express predominantly IL-4, IDEC induce Th2 cells to express predominantly IFN-γ [30]. The findings of a relatively new cutaneous DC subset, plasmacytoid (pDC) further suggest DC play an important role in AD. This subset is found to be deficient in AD skin, as compared to those in psoriasis and contact dermatitis. pDC are important producers of the anti-viral cytokines IFN-α and IFN-β, and it is believed that its absence in AD lesions may promote AD patients more susceptible to viral infections [31].

Genetics

Recent research findings suggested genetics play a critical role in maintaining the proper function of the skin barrier. Up to 60% European AD patients demonstrated either single or double-allele mutations in *FLG*, suggesting mutations in the gene of filaggrin (*FLG*) is a key player in contributing to the pathogenesis of AD [32-34]. Decreased in *FLG* expression will lead to a decrease in keratohyalin granules, causing a disruption of the stratum granulosum and a defect in the differentiation and growth of a normal SC structure [35, 36]. Other genetic pathways are also well known to be implicated in the pathogenesis of AD. For example, mutated *SPINK5* in crucial in contributing to Netherton Syndrome, increasing the susceptibility to AD [37-39].

Other Environmental Factors

There are other environmental factors which may contribute to the pathogenesis pf AD. For example, weather humidity can accelerate transepidermal water loss (TEWL) in AD and allowing further inflammatory cytokines infiltration [40]. Psychological factors such as stress may also inhibit the synthesis of the structural molecules and hydrophobic barriers of SC including ceramides, cholesterols, and free fatty acids [17]. These triggers vary among individuals immunologically, and can include foods, airborne allergens, irritants and contactants, hormones, stress, climate, and microorganisms etc. [2].

Prognosis

Due to the complexity of the disorder, the management of AD always presents a great challenge to all clinicians. Generally, AD has a good prognosis. Nevertheless, it can sometimes cause significant morbidity, as its signs and symptoms can significantly affect the quality of lives of affected children and families, thereby disrupting family life and causing sleep deprivation [7, 8]. Current therapeutic approaches of AD often focuses on symptomatic relief and control rather than cure [41], and the long-term treatment objectives for AD are confined to reducing the clinical manifestations, minimizing relapses, and improving the disease course. These approaches comprise basic skin care for cutaneous and liberal use of emollients for rehydration, intermittent application of anti-inflammatory therapy for acute flares, as well as refraining from triggering factors [42, 43].

CURRENT TREATMENT OPTIONS

Basic Topical Therapy with Emollients in Atopic Dermatitis

Due to the disruption in the epidermal barrier function of the skin of AD patients, it is important to apply topical applications which could effectively improve the SC moisture to stabilize the reduced epidermal barrier function. There are numerous emollient products being marketed to treat eczema, but not all of them are effective. Hon et al. had previously provided a thorough review summarizing current available data on a number of moisturizers/emollients and putting their claimed ingredients together in comparison to provide clinical-based evidence and objective options for considering the most appropriate emollient [44]. In general, these common active ingredients in emollients include petroleum products, glycerin, fatty acids and plant oils. While most of these moisturizers demonstrate beneficial effects, there was however no evidence which suggest one is more superior to another. It would therefore be important for physicians to provide evidence-based information for the different emollients on the patients [44].

Topical Corticosteroids

Cortisol, the physiologically occurring adrenal steroid, together with its derivatives glucocorticosteroids, are the most widely used topical preparations in dermatology. It was firstly discovered by Hench et al. in 1950 as a systemically administered adrenal cortical hormone (17-hydroxy11-dehydrorcorticosterone, compound E) with therapeutic values, which in turn lead to their receipt of Nobel Prizes [45, 46]. Two years later,

Sulzberger and Witten introduced the use of cortisol topically as hydrocortisone, marking a major pharmacologic breakthrough in dermatotherapy. Since then hydrocortisone has served as a common treatment for AD [47].

Corticosteroid contributes its effect by regulation of the inflammatory cascade in AD. There are three main mechanism of actions by which it acts: vasoconstriction, anti-inflammatory effects, and anti-proliferative effects [10]. While topically on the skin, corticosteroids can modify the functions of epidermal and dermal cells, and leukocytes involved in the proliferation and inflammatory action. They can then further pass through the cell membrane to react with receptor proteins to form a steroid-receptor complex, which in turn bind to DNA, thereby changing mRNA transcription and inhibiting inflammatory cytokines synthesis such as IL-1. Corticosteroids can also stimulate the production of lipocortin, a glycoprotein which is responsible for inhibiting the activity of phospholipase A2, which releases arachidonic acid, the precursor of prostanoids and leukotrienes from phospholipids [48]. Further studies of the mechanism of action of corticosteroids are warranted to provide further insight on how corticosteroids work, and provide fundamental information that is essential for the development of novel non-steroidal anti-inflammatory drugs [10].

Despite the potent therapeutic values of corticosteroids, they also come with undesirable side effects with prolonged or over dosage use. These effects had become increasingly evident and well known to the public. Nevertheless, these consequences had been overestimated overtime, thereby causing many AD patients to reject corticosteroid treatment entirely. Most of the fear on the unwanted effects of side effects of corticosteroid are unnecessary and can be avoided should corticosteroid be applied cautiously and in a sensible manner. Furthermore, depending on the course of administration, the degree of side effects of topical corticosteroid application can differ. Short-term application is generally associated with less side effects while the unwanted effects are more likely to be associated with prolonged or high-dose usage.

Table 1. Representative preparations of topical corticosteroid classified in groups

Potency	Class	Topical corticosteroid	Formulation
Ultra high	I	Clobetasol propionate	Cream, 0.05%
		Diflorasone diacetate	Ointment, 0.05%
High	II	Amcinonide	Ointment, 0.1%
		Betamethasone dipropionat	Ointment, 0.05%
		Desoximetasone	Cream or ointment, 0.025%
		Fluocinonide	Cream, ointment or gel, 0.05%
		Halcinonide	Cream, 0.1%
	III	Betamethasone dipropionate	Cream, 0.05%
		Betamethasone valerate	Ointment, 0.1%
		Diflorasone diacetate	Cream, 0.05%
		Triamcinolone acetonide	Ointment, 0.1%
Moderate	IV	Desoximetasone	Cream, 0.05%
		Fluocinolone acetonide	Ointment, 0.025%
		Fludroxycortide	Ointment, 0.05%
		Hydrocortisone valerate	Ointment, 0.2%
		Triamcinolone acetonide	Cream, 0.1%
	V	Betamethasone dipropionate	Lotion, 0.02%
		Betamethasone valerate	Cream, 0.1%
		Fluocinolone acetonide	Cream, 0.025%
		Fludroxycortide	Cream, 0.05%
		Hydrocortisone butyrate	Cream, 0.1%
		Hydrocortisone valerate	Cream, 0.2%
		Triamcinolone acetonide	Lotion, 0.1%
Low	VI	Betamethasone valerate	Lotion, 0.05%
		Desonide	Cream, 0.05%
		Fluocinolone acetonide	Solution, 0.01%
	VII	Dexamethasone sodium	Cream, 0.1%
		phosphate	Cream, 1%
		Hydrocortisone acetate	Cream, 0.25%
		Methylprednisolone acetate	

Modified from WHO.

According to World Health Organization (WHO), topical corticosteroids can be classified into different classes according to their potency [49]. There are four groups consisting of seven class: ultra-high-potency (Class I); high-potency (Class II and III); moderate potency (Class

IV and V); and moderate potency (Class VI and VII). Table 1 shows the different commercially available topical corticosteroids tabled in accordance to their class and potency. Class I topical corticosteroids are the most potent and Class VII are the least potent adapted from WHO. Efficacy and side-effects are greatest with the Class I ultra-high-potency preparations which should only be used for limited time periods (2-3 weeks) [49].

In the face of the efficacy observed in the usage of topical corticosteroid, systemic corticosteroids are generally not recommended. According to the clinical practice guidelines and position statements concerning the management of AD, the use of systemic corticosteroids including prednisone, hydrocortisone and celestone are discouraged with only very limited exceptions since systemic application would hinder increased risk of more severe side-effects or rebound flares after discontinuation despite their rapid clearing of AD.

Antihistamines

As discussed earlier, T cell activation is one of the key events observed in AD. Activated T cells can secrete histamine releasing factor contributing to the itching behavior in AD patients [50]. Being the central primary and most distressing symptom, pharmaceuticals that is able to manage or ease such uncomfortable allergic reaction is of great importance. Antihistamines has long been used as an additional therapy to control itchiness. Numerous studies suggested IgE-mediated reactions are an aggravating factor in the majority of AD patients and that both an increase of mast cells and dermal histamine have been observed in atopic dermatitis [10]. Antihistamine works to reduce itchiness by blocking the action of histamine on its receptors in the skin to avoid the pruritic histamine effects [16, 51].

The earliest use of antihistamine can be traced back to 1950, when the first generation of antihistamine drugs were marketed. Although this first generation antihistamine may help to reduce itchiness, side effects exist include dry mouth, sedation and impaired cognitive function [10].

Interestingly, the use of these first generation and yet sedative antihistamine are favored by many doctors with the insight that sedative effect could reduce the impulse of the patients to scratch since AD patients tend to damage their skin through uncontrolled scratching behavior causing sleep deprivation [10].

The newer second generation antihistamine are considered less or even non-sedative without the side effects of dry mouth. Examples of these newer generation antihistamine include azelastine, cetirizine, desoxyloratadine, ebastine and fexofenadine levocetirizine. These agents are less lipophilic and are less likely to penetrate into the central nervous system (CNS) [10]. These agents also possess a higher and more specific binding to the H1-receptor, and less non-specific binding to the cholinergic receptors. Contradictive comments and debates arise regarding the efficacy of these two generations of antihistamine. Further supportive clinical studies are required to provide evidence based information on the efficacy of antihistamine agents on AD patients.

Systemic Immunomodulators

Most patients with AD have mild to moderate disease. However, a subpopulation of patients may develop more severe symptoms including extensive area of skin lesions and persistent itchiness which significantly affect the patient's quality of life either physically or emotionally. These patients with severe AD generally do not respond well to first-line topical therapies, and hence more intensive or systematic therapies such as immunomodulators may be required. Examples of these common immunosuppressant medications are cyclosporine, methotrexate, azathioprine, and mycophenolate mofetil [16]. Similar to corticosteroids, the course of treatment such as dosage, frequency and duration will need to be prescribed by physician.

Cyclosporine

Cyclosporine was firstly used in 1991 [17]. It is a polypeptide of fungal origin which acts by binding to cyclophilin of lymphocytes to inhibit calcineurin, thereby blocking activated T cells for IL-2 and other inflammatory cytokines production [16, 17, 51]. Doses of cyclosporine used will depend on factors such as age, disease severity, medical comorbidities, and tolerability of the patient [17]. Cyclosporine has proven to be safe and efficacious in general. However, increased risk of adverse effects include kidney toxicity, hypertension and even lymphoma and skin cancer are observed at high dose usage [16].

Mycophenolate Mofetil

Oral mycophenolate mofetil is generally considered an effective and well-tolerated drug for treating severe AE. It is an immunosuppressant which inhibits inosine monophosphate dehydrogenase to block purine synthesis selectively in T cells and B cells [17]. Currently FDA only approved its usage in organ transplantation, and hence its off-label use in patients with severe AD will need to adhere strictly in accordance to physician's instructions [16, 17].

Methotrexate

Methotrexate are immunosuppressants that work by inhibiting the synthesis of DNA and RNA to slow down the metabolism of new cells. It can also inhibit enzymes involved in purine metabolism and cause accumulation of adenosine which in turn inhibit T-cell activation. Common side effects include nausea, GI symptoms, and fatigue. Rarely, yet more serious side effects include bone marrow suppression, pulmonary fibrosis or even hepatotoxicity. Caution will need to be considered when being prescribed to patients with asthma, chronic cough, or other pulmonary disease. A complete pulmonary evaluation is suggested prior to initiating therapy in these patients [17].

OTHER THERAPIES

Anti-Microbial Therapy

Patients with AD often exhibit skins colonize with microbes such as *Staphylococcus aureus* (*S. aureus*). These infectious pathogens also play a significant role in provoking further immuno reaction in AD patients [10]. Clinically, *S. aureus* was found in approximately 90% of the patients whom had developed chronic AD lichenified plaques [52]. Interestingly, the density of *S. aureus* tends to increase with the clinical severity of the atopic eczema lesions [51]. It is suggested that the dryness of eczematous skin is due to deficiency in certain inhibitory fatty acid, thereby favoring the growth and adherence of the bacteria to skin cells [51, 52]. Other speculated that the pathogenic role of *S. aureus* in AD could be due to a direct chemical irritation, a non-specific reaction of the protein A component of the bacterium with immune cells which produces super antigens that is capable of stimulating of T-lymphocyte production, leading to the widespread activation of eczematous lesions. The pathogenic role of *S. aureus* has led to the use of many antimicrobial compounds such as oral antibiotics against *S. aureus*, or topically applied antibiotics, and antiseptic agents applied directly or by mixing with emollients applied directly to the skin or during bath [51]. Not only bacterial, but also viral and fungal superinfections are well known risk factors causing acute and severe disease exacerbation. Therefore, antimicrobial therapy is an important treatment component in the management of AE [10]. Nevertheless, deliberate or general use of antimicrobials are not recommended due to the emergence of resistant organisms and the sensitizing potential of many antibiotic preparations.

Traditional Chinese Medicine (TCM)

Traditional Chinese Medicine has a long history in the treatment of AD. While being considered as an allergy disorder in Western medicine, according to the TCM theory, AD is caused by accumulation of dampness and heat within the body, causing spleen weakness and stagnation of phlegm. The recurrent and chronic nature of AD can injure Yin and blood and generate dryness Chinese herbal decoctions prescribed predominately focus on using herbs which could clear heat, remove dampness and phlegm, and ability to tonify the spleen [53].

Effects of TCM decoctions on AD had also been scientifically studied in evidence-based clinical trials. Sheena et al. carried out two clinical trial studies studying the efficacy of TCM decoctions compromising Saposhnikoviae Radix, Potentilla chinensis Herba, Akebiae Caulis, Rehmanniae Radix, Moutan Cortex, Lophatheri Herba, Dictamni Cortex, Tribuli Fructus, Glycyrrhiza Radix, Schizonepetae Herba in children and adults. Both of which demonstrated significant beneficial effects of TCM treatment compared with placebo, highlighting a promising treatment of atopic eczema [51]. Hon et al. evaluated the effects of another TCM deocoction PentaHerbs formula (PHF) in several clinical studies. PentaHerbs formula (PHF) is a traditional Chinese herb concoction which contains Cortex Moutan, the dried root bark of Paeonia suffruticosa Andr. (Ranunculaceae), Cortex Phellodendri, the dried bark of Phellodendron chinensis Schneid. (Rutaceae), Flos Lonicerae, the dried flower of Lonicera japonica Thunb. (Capri-foliaceae), Herba Menthae, the dried aerial part of Mentha haplocalyx Briq. (Labiatae) and Rhizoma Atractylodis, the dried rhizome of Atractylodes lancea (Thunb.) DC. (Compositae) in the ratio of 2:2:2:1:2 [54]. Upon trials in these several clinical studies, it was concluded that PHF is well tolerated and efficacious in improving the quality of life in children. It could also reduce the amount of topical corticosteroid used in children with moderate-to-severe AD [55-58]. Interestingly, *in vitro* mechanistic study suggested that PHF could suppress inflammatory mediators release from mast cells, of which Cortex Montan and Herba Menthae were the two most effective herbs in suppressing mast cell mediator release out of the five herbs in the formulation [54].

Nevertheless, the beneficial effects of TCM on AD have not been consistently demonstrated. A limited number of clinical trials failed to show convincing results [59]. Efficacy of TCM on AD will need to depend on the herbs used, as not every herbs would exert beneficial effects. Adverse effects of TCM are not uncommon and have been previously reported, with liver damage as the most commonly seen unfavorable side effects. As the use of TCM has become increasingly popular with AD, evaluation of the efficacy of TCM using the modern scientific platform to provide a more in depth investigation on the efficacy of TCM from *in vitro* mechanistic studies to *in vivo* efficacy, followed by large scale and properly designed clinical studies with good clinical practice are warranted to provide more conclusive and evidence-based data on their clinical application.

CONCLUSION

The complexity of the pathophysiology of AD has led to difficulties in finding the cure for AD. Current management of AD rely on symptomic management which involves the long-term use of topical corticosteroid, immunomodulators, anti-microbial agents or combination of therapies to combat the variety of pathologic processes. These treatments can be associated with adverse events or even development of drug tolerance. While alternative therapies such as TCM are widely adapted by patients particularly in Asia, their beneficial effects or efficacy have not been consistently demonstrated. Such concern is increased by the fact that there is a lack of standardization of TCM. Providing scientific explanations on clinical efficacies of TCM are of great importance in moving forward to open up more innovative treatment options for such complicated disorder.

REFERENCES

[1] Kamer B., Pasowska R., Dolka E., Blomberg A., Rotsztejn H., Prevalence of atopic dermatitis in infants during the first six months of life: authors' observations, *Postepy Dermatol Alergol* 30(5) (2013) 277-81.

[2] Abramovits W., Atopic dermatitis, *J Am Acad Dermatol* 53(1 Suppl 1) (2005) S86-93.

[3] Hulshof L., Overbeek S. A., Wyllie A. L., Chu M., Bogaert D., de Jager W., Knippels L. M. J., Sanders E. A. M., van Aalderen W. M. C., Garssen J., Van't Land B., Sprikkelman A. B., Clinical Study, Exploring Immune Development in Infants With Moderate to Severe Atopic Dermatitis, *Front Immunol* 9 (2018) 630.

[4] Leung D. Y., Bieber T., Atopic dermatitis, *Lancet* 361(9352) (2003) 151-60.

[5] Oszukowska M., Michalak I., Gutfreund K., Bienias W., Matych M., Szewczyk A., Kaszuba A., Role of primary and secondary prevention in atopic dermatitis, *Postepy Dermatol Alergol* 32(6) (2015) 409-20.

[6] Williams H. C., Is the prevalence of atopic dermatitis increasing?, *Clin Exp Dermatol* 17(6) (1992) 385-91.

[7] Carroll C. L., Balkrishnan R., Feldman S. R., Fleischer A. B., Jr., Manuel J. C., The burden of atopic dermatitis: impact on the patient, family, and society, *Pediatr Dermatol* 22(3) (2005) 192-9.

[8] Watson W., Kapur S., Atopic dermatitis, Allergy Asthma *Clin Immunol* 7 Suppl 1 (2011) S4.

[9] Engman M. F., Weiss R. S., Engman M. E., Eczema and environment, *Med Clin North Am* 20 (1936) 651-63.

[10] Ring J., Przybilla B., Ruzicka T., *Handbook of atopic eczema*, Second Edition ed., Springer-Verlag Berlin Heidelberg New York, Germany, 2006.

[11] Hanifin J. M., Rajka, G. Diagnostic features of atopic dermatitis, *Acta Derm Venereol* (Stockh) Suppl 92 (1980) 44 –47.

[12] Boothe W. David, Tarbox J. A., Tarbox M. B., Atopic Dermatitis: Pathophysiology, *Adv Exp Med Biol* 1027 (2017) 21-37.

[13] Kim J., Kim B. E., Leung D. Y. M., Pathophysiology of atopic dermatitis: Clinical implications, *Allergy Asthma Proc* 40(2) (2019) 84-92.

[14] Lowe A. J., Leung D. Y. M., Tang M. L. K., Su J. C., Allen K. J., The skin as a target for prevention of the atopic march, *Ann Allergy Asthma Immunol* 120(2) (2018) 145-151.

[15] Dharmage S. C., Lowe A. J., Matheson M. C., Burgess J. A., Allen K. J., Abramson M. J., Atopic dermatitis and the atopic march revisited, *Allergy* 69(1) (2014) 17-27.

[16] Van Bever H. A., MarcieMom A., Living with eczema: mom asks, doc answers! WSPC; 1st edition (2014).

[17] Fortson E. A., Feldman S. R., Strowd L. C., *Management of Atopic Dermatitis - Methods and Challenges*, Springer International Publishing, Switzerland, 2017.

[18] Seidenari S., Giusti G., Objective assessment of the skin of children affected by atopic dermatitis: a study of pH, capacitance and TEWL in eczematous and clinically uninvolved skin, *Acta Derm Venereol* 75(6) (1995) 429-33.

[19] Thyssen J. P., Kezic S., Causes of epidermal filaggrin reduction and their role in the pathogenesis of atopic dermatitis, *J Allergy Clin Immunol* 134(4) (2014) 792-9.

[20] Egawa, G., K. Kabashima, Barrier dysfunction in the skin allergy, *Allergol Int* 67(1) (2018) 3-11.

[21] Howell M. D., Kim B. E., Gao P., Grant A. V., Boguniewicz M., DeBenedetto A., Schneider L., Beck L. A., Barnes K. C., Leung D. Y., Cytokine modulation of atopic dermatitis filaggrin skin expression, *J Allergy Clin Immunol* 124(3 Suppl 2) (2009) R7-R12.

[22] Leonardi S., Rotolo N., Vitaliti G., Spicuzza L., La Rosa M., IgE values and T-lymphocyte subsets in children with atopic eczema/dermatitis syndrome, *Allergy Asthma Proc* 28(5) (2007) 529-34.

[23] Gavrilova T., Immune Dysregulation in the Pathogenesis of Atopic Dermatitis, *Dermatitis* 29(2) (2018) 57-62.

[24] Leung D. Y., New insights into atopic dermatitis: role of skin barrier and immune dysregulation, *Allergol Int* 62(2) (2013) 151-61.

[25] Gittler J. K., Shemer A., Suarez-Farinas M., Fuentes-Duculan J., Gulewicz K. J., Wang C. Q., Mitsui H., Cardinale I., de Guzman Strong C., Krueger J. G., Guttman-Yassky E., Progressive activation of T(H)2/T(H)22 cytokines and selective epidermal proteins characterizes acute and chronic atopic dermatitis, *J Allergy Clin Immunol* 130(6) (2012) 1344-54.

[26] Cornelissen C., Marquardt Y., Czaja K., Wenzel J., Frank J., Luscher-Firzlaff J., Luscher B., Baron J. M., IL-31 regulates differentiation and filaggrin expression in human organotypic skin models, *J Allergy Clin Immunol* 129(2) (2012) 426-33, 433 e1-8.

[27] Herrick C. A., Xu L., McKenzie A. N., Tigelaar R. E., Bottomly K., IL-13 is necessary, not simply sufficient, for epicutaneously induced Th2 responses to soluble protein antigen, *J Immunol* 170(5) (2003) 2488-95.

[28] Purwar R., Werfel T., Wittmann M., IL-13-stimulated human keratinocytes preferentially attract CD4+CCR4+ T cells: possible role in atopic dermatitis, *J Invest Dermatol* 126(5) (2006) 1043-51.

[29] Ong P. Y., Leung D. Y., Immune dysregulation in atopic dermatitis, *Curr Allergy Asthma Rep* 6(5) (2006) 384-9.

[30] Novak N., Valenta R., Bohle B., Laffer S., Haberstok J., Kraft S., Bieber T., FcepsilonRI engagement of Langerhans cell-like dendritic cells and inflammatory dendritic epidermal cell-like dendritic cells induces chemotactic signals and different T-cell phenotypes in vitro, *J Allergy Clin Immunol* 113(5) (2004) 949-57.

[31] Wollenberg A., Wagner M., Gunther S., Towarowski A., Tuma E., Moderer M., Rothenfusser S., Wetzel S., Endres S., Hartmann G., Plasmacytoid dendritic cells: a new cutaneous dendritic cell subset with distinct role in inflammatory skin diseases, *J Invest Dermatol* 119(5) (2002) 1096-102.

[32] Elias P. M., Schmuth M., Abnormal skin barrier in the etiopathogenesis of atopic dermatitis, *Curr Allergy Asthma Rep* 9(4) (2009) 265-72.

[33] McAleer M. A., Irvine A. D., The multifunctional role of filaggrin in allergic skin disease, *J Allergy Clin Immunol* 131(2) (2013) 280-91.

[34] Palmer C. N., Irvine A. D., Terron-Kwiatkowski A., Zhao Y., Liao H., Lee S. P., Goudie D. R., Sandilands A., Campbell L. E., Smith F. J., O'Regan G. M., Watson R. M., Cecil J. E., Bale S. J., Compton J. G., DiGiovanna J. J., Fleckman P., Lewis-Jones S., Arseculeratne G., Sergeant A., Munro C. S., Houate B. El, McElreavey K., L Halkjaer.B., Bisgaard H., Mukhopadhyay S., McLean W. H., Common loss-of-function variants of the epidermal barrier protein filaggrin are a major predisposing factor for atopic dermatitis, *Nat Genet* 38(4) (2006) 441-6.

[35] Fleckman P., Brumbaugh S., Absence of the granular layer and keratohyalin define a morphologically distinct subset of individuals with ichthyosis vulgaris, *Exp Dermatol* 11(4) (2002) 327-36.

[36] Scharschmidt T. C., Man M. Q., Hatano Y., Crumrine D., Gunathilake R., Sundberg J. P., Silva K. A., Mauro T. M., Hupe M., Cho, Wu S. Y., Celli A., Schmuth M., Feingold K. R., Elias P. M., Filaggrin deficiency confers a paracellular barrier abnormality that reduces inflammatory thresholds to irritants and haptens, *J Allergy Clin Immunol* 124(3) (2009) 496-506, 506 e1-6.

[37] Kato A., Fukai K., Oiso N., Hosomi N., Murakami T., Ishii M., Association of SPINK5 gene polymorphisms with atopic dermatitis in the Japanese population, *Br J Dermatol* 148(4) (2003) 665-9.

[38] Zhao L. P., Di Z., Zhang L., Wang L., Ma L., Lv Y., Hong Y., Wei H., Chen H. D., Gao X. H., Association of SPINK5 gene polymorphisms with atopic dermatitis in Northeast China, *J Eur Acad Dermatol Venereol* 26(5) (2012) 572-7.

[39] Walley A. J., Chavanas S., Moffatt M. F., Esnouf R. M., Ubhi B., Lawrence R., Wong K., Abecasis G. R., Jones E. Y., Harper J. I., Hovnanian A., Cookson W. O., Gene polymorphism in Netherton and common atopic disease, *Nat Genet* 29(2) (2001) 175-8.

[40] Sato J., Denda M., Chang S., Elias P. M., Feingold K. R., Abrupt decreases in environmental humidity induce abnormalities in

permeability barrier homeostasis, *J Invest Dermatol* 119(4) (2002) 900-4.

[41] Flohr C., Mann J., New approaches to the prevention of childhood atopic dermatitis, *Allergy* 69(1) (2014) 56-61.

[42] Yeung C. K., Chan H. H. L., Recent Advances in Childhood Atopic Dermatitis, *HK J Paediatr* (New Series) 12 (2007) 270-282.

[43] Wollenberg A., Ehmann L. M., Long term treatment concepts and proactive therapy for atopic eczema, *Ann Dermatol* 24(3) (2012) 253-60.

[44] Hon K. L., Kung J. S. C., Ng W. G. G., Leung T. F., Emollient treatment of atopic dermatitis: latest evidence and clinical considerations, *Drugs Context* 7 (2018) 212530.

[45] Hench P. S., Kendall E. C., Slocumb C. H., Polley H. F., The effect of a hormone of the adrenal cortex (17-hydroxy-11-dehydrocorticosterone: compound E) and of pituitary adrenocortical hormone in arthritis: preliminary report, *Ann Rheum Dis* 8(2) (1949) 97-104.

[46] Kaiser H., Kley H. K., *Cortisontherapie: Corticoide in Klinik und Praxi*, 11th ed., Thieme, Stuttgart, 2002.

[47] Sulzberger M. B., Witten V. H., The effect of topically applied compound F in selected dermatoses, *J Invest Dermatol* 19(2) (1952) 101-2.

[48] Kragballe K., Topical corticosteroids: mechanisms of action, *Acta Derm Venereol Suppl* (Stockh) 151 (1989) 7-10; discussion 47-52.

[49] W.H. Organization, *WHO model prescribing information: drugs used in skin diseases*, Geneva: World Health Organization, Switzerland, 1997.

[50] Kashiwakura J. I., Ando T., Kawakami T., Role of Histamine-releasing Factor in Allergic Inflammatory Reactions, *Yakugaku Zasshi* 137(5) (2017) 517-521.

[51] Hoare C., A. Po L i Wan, Williams H., Systematic review of treatments for atopic eczema, *Health Technol Assess* 4(37) (2000) 1-191.

[52] Leyden J. J., Marples R. R., Kligman A. M., *Staphylococcus aureus* in the lesions of atopic dermatitis, *Br J Dermatol* 90(5) (1974) 525-30.

[53] Lu C., Jin X., Wu D., Zhu S., Liu Tuina for treatment of atopic eczema in children under 14 years: A systematic review of randomized controlled trials, *Journal of Tradditional Chinese Medical Sciences,* 6(1) (2019) 13-25.

[54] Chan B. C., Hon K. L., Leung P. C., Sam S. W., Fung K. P., Lee M. Y., Lau H. Y., Traditional Chinese medicine for atopic eczema: PentaHerbs formula suppresses inflammatory mediators release from mast cells, *J Ethnopharmacol* 120(1) (2008) 85-91.

[55] Hon K. L., Leung T. F., Wong Y., Lam W. K., Guan D. Q., Ma K. C., Sung Y. T., Fok T. F., Leung P. C., A pentaherbs capsule as a treatment option for atopic dermatitis in children: an open-labeled case series, *Am J Chin Med* 32(6) (2004) 941-50.

[56] Hon K. L., Leung T. F., Ng P. C., Lam M. C., Kam W. Y., Wong K. Y., Lee K. C., Sung Y. T., Cheng K. F., Fok T. F., Fung K. P., Leung P.C., Efficacy and tolerability of a Chinese herbal medicine concoction for treatment of atopic dermatitis: a randomized, double-blind, placebo-controlled study, *Br J Dermatol* 157(2) (2007) 357-63.

[57] Leung T. F., Wong K. Y., Wong C. K., Fung K. P., Lam C. W., Fok T. F., Leung P. C., Hon K. L., In vitro and clinical immunomodulatory effects of a novel Pentaherbs concoction for atopic dermatitis, *Br J Dermatol* 158(6) (2008) 1216-23.

[58] Hon K. L., Lo W., Cheng W. K., Leung T. F., Chow C. M., Lau C. B., Fok T. F., Ng P. C., Leung P. C., Prospective self-controlled trial of the efficacy and tolerability of a herbal syrup for young children with eczema, *J Dermatolog Treat* 23(2) (2012) 116-21.

[59] Hon K. L., Chan B. C., Leung P. C., Chinese herbal medicine research in eczema treatment, *Chin Med* 6 (2011) 17.

In: Atopic Dermatitis
Editor: Andreas Maur
ISBN: 978-1-53618-520-1

Chapter 4

EMERGING THERAPIES FOR ATOPIC DERMATITIS

***Ge Peng*[1,2] *and François Niyonsaba*[2,3,*]**

[1]Department of Dermatology and Allergology, Juntendo University Graduate School of Medicine, Tokyo, Japan

[2]Atopy (Allergy) Research Center, Juntendo University Graduate School of Medicine, Tokyo, Japan

[3]Faculty of International Liberal Arts, Juntendo University, Tokyo, Japan

ABSTRACT

Atopic dermatitis (AD) is a common chronic, pruritic, inflammatory dermatosis that affects the population worldwide. AD is primarily characterized by skin barrier dysfunction and is mediated by a cutaneous immune response. To date, the primary therapy for AD inflammation is still the use of topical corticosteroids, while severe refractory and inadequately controlled AD cases are treated with systemic immune-

* Corresponding Author's E-mail: francois@juntendo.ac.jp.

suppressive medications. Growing knowledge of the pathogenesis of AD has allowed recent development of more targeted topical and systemic therapies by supplementing barrier function, suppressing inflammation or inhibiting elevated T helper (Th) 2 cytokines (interleukin (IL)-4, IL-5, IL-13, IL-33, thymic stromal lymphopoietin and their receptors) or Th22/Th17 cytokines. In addition, there are also other emerging therapies, such as inhibitors of phosphodiesterase, Janus kinase, immunoglobulin E and histamine, and antipruritic agents. Besides, because dysbiosis in the skin microbiome enables *Staphylococcus aureus* colonization, which exacerbates inflammation in AD, the transplantation of commensal strains and anti-staphylococcal treatment targeting *Staphylococcus aureus* are also promising therapies under investigation. This chapter provides insight into various emerging therapies along with currently approved treatments for AD.

Keywords: atopic dermatitis, biologics, inhibitors, therapy, treatments

ABBREVIATIONS

AD:	atopic dermatitis;
AhR:	aryl hydrocarbon receptor;
EASI:	Eczema Area and Severity Index;
FDA:	Food and Drug Administration;
FLG:	filaggrin;
H4R:	histamine receptor type 4;
IGA:	Investigator's Global Assessment;
IL:	interleukin;
ILC2:	group 2 innate lymphoid cell;
JAK:	Janus kinase;
PDE4:	phosphodiesterase 4;
S. aureus	*Staphylococcus aureus*;
TCI:	topical calcineurin inhibitor;
TCS:	topical corticosteroid;
Th:	helper T cell;
TSLP:	thymic stromal lymphopoietin.

1. INTRODUCTION

Atopic dermatitis (AD), also known as atopic eczema, is a common chronic, pruritic, inflammatory dermatosis affecting over 200 million patients worldwide [1-3]. The first-line therapy for mild AD for decades has been topical corticosteroids (TCSs). However, persistent application of TCSs can result in adverse effects varying from barely perceptible, fully reversible thinning, to irreversible telangiectasia and striae distensae [4]. Systemic immunosuppressive medications (cyclosporine, methotrexate, mycophenolate mofetil, short-term use of systemic corticosteroids) can be used for moderate-to-severe AD cases where TCSs are ineffective. However, systemic treatments should be used only for a short time because they have the risk of widely compromising immune function [5, 6]. Recently, topical calcineurin inhibitors (TCIs) have been recommended as a second-line therapy. TCIs can be repeatedly used in patients with persistent AD on lesional sites where the side effects caused by TCSs may easily develop. Although TCIs have fewer side effects than TCSs, TCIs are reported to cause burning of the skin and have received a "black box" warning from the Food and Drug Administration (FDA) because of a possible association with nonmelanoma skin cancer and lymphoma development [7, 8].

Although there are continuing debates about the primary events and key drivers of AD pathogenesis [9], it is now clear that the dysregulation of the skin barrier function, immune system and skin microbiota is closely involved in the development of AD [10]. In addition, there is growing interest in the underlying mechanisms of itching with the correlation of inflammatory mediators and the peripheral and central nervous systems [11]. In the past decade, emerging understanding of key factors involved in AD pathogenesis has yielded great success in the development of new therapeutic options through improving the cutaneous barrier, inhibiting overactivated immune pathways, regulating skin dysbiosis, and reducing itching.

This chapter provides insight into approved treatments and emerging therapies for AD in the following sections: (1) barrier repair therapy; (2)

therapy targeting type 2 immunity; (3) therapy targeting other helper T cell pathways; (4) broad-targeting therapy; (5) antipruritic agents and (6) the regulation of the skin microbiome. We believe that a deep understanding of the pathogenesis of AD will lead to further improvements in the prevention and management of this chronic skin disorder.

2. Barrier Repair Therapy

AD exhibits prominent barrier defects due to various factors, such as the disruption of the stratum corneum; mutations in corneocyte structural proteins, such as filaggrin (FLG); abnormal lipid organization; and a deficiency of antimicrobial peptides (AMPs) [12]. Although topical application of moisturizers has long been the basic requirement for barrier repair of AD, many more studies have focused on different specific compositions to target the abovementioned defective factors, thereby improving the skin barrier. Recently, VTP-38543, a liver X receptor (LXR)-selective agonist, was developed to improve barrier function and decrease inflammation in damaged skin tissue. In preclinical studies, ligand-mediated activation of LXRs resulted in keratinocyte differentiation, the induction of lipid synthesis and cholesterol transport, and decreased inflammation in human macrophages and in mouse models of dermatitis [13]. Topical use of VTP-38543 has been applied to adult patients with mild-to-moderate AD in a phase I/II trial, in which this formulation significantly increased the mRNA expression of FLG and lipids and reduced keratin 16, an epidermal hyperplasia marker [14].

In healthy skin, FLG is degraded by the cysteine peptidase caspase-14 into natural moisturizing factors (NMFs), including free amino acids, pyrrolidine carboxylic acid, and urocanic acid (UCA) [15], which provide moisture retention and maintain the acidic pH of the skin, thereby strengthening the stratum corneum barrier. Patients with AD who carry FLG mutations have fewer NMFs than their counterparts lacking these mutations [16-18]. A cis-UCA emulsion cream improved skin barrier function and suppressed inflammation in human skin. The topical application of this cream improved the Eczema Area Severity Index (EASI) score from baseline for patients with AD in a randomized phase I/IIa trial, without causing any remarkable adverse effects [19].

Table 1. Interventional clinical trials with novel barrier repair therapies in atopic dermatitis

Target	Treatment	Population/ severity	Phase of current development/ status	NCT No.	Route
Liver X receptor	VTP-38543	18-65y/MM	I/II/completed	NCT02655679	Topical
	ALX 101	>12y/Mo	II/active, not recruiting	NCT03859986	Topical
		>12y/Mo	II/completed	NCT03175354	Topical
DGLA	DS107	>18y/MS	IIb/completed	NCT02864498	Oral
		>18y/MS	II/recruiting	NCT03817190	Oral
		>18y/MM	IIb/completed	NCT02925793	Topical
	DS107E	18-65y/MS	II/completed	NCT03676036	Topical
		3-12M/MS	II/completed	NCT03676933	Topical
	DS107G	>18y/MS	II/completed	NCT02211417	Oral
Cri-UCA	Cis-UCA cream	>18y/MM	I/IIa/completed	NCT01320579	Topical
Unknown	EpiCeram	3m-12y/Mo	IV/completed	NCT00828412	Topical
Unknown	Atopiclair	2-17y/MM	IV/completed	NCT01093469	Topical
		18-65y/MM	NA/completed	NCT01079897	Topical
Unknown	BRT-FC -83C	18-0y/MM	II/completed	NCT00883311	Topical
Unknown	PDI-192	3m-17y/MM	II/completed	NCT01826461	Topical
Unknown	IDP-124	>2y/MS	III/recruiting	NCT03002571	Topical
		>2y/MS	III/recruiting	NCT03058783	Topical
Unknown	TLA Treatment	4-16y/MS	NA/recruiting	NCT03795506	External device
AMP	Omiganan/ CLS 001/ MBI 226	18-65y/MS	II/completed	NCT03091426	Topical
		18-65y/MS	II/completed	NCT02456480	Topical
	DPK-060	18-65y/MMS	I/II/completed	NCT01522391	Topical

NA: not applicable; MM: mild-to-moderate; Mo: moderate; MS: moderate-to-severe; MMS: mild, moderate and severe; AMP: antimicrobial peptide; DGLA: dihomo gamma linolenic acid; TLA: nocturnal temperature-controlled laminar airflow; UCA: urocanic acid.

AMPs, the key molecules in the cutaneous immune system, not only exhibit broad-spectrum antimicrobial activities but also have important immunomodulatory functions, including the regulation of inflammatory responses, the control of the production of various cytokines/chemokines, the promotion of cell proliferation and migration, the regulation of itching and the improvement of skin barrier function [20-22]. To date, several topical antimicrobial agents, including omiganan (a synthetic derivative based on bovine neutrophil indolicidin) and DPK-060 (derived from the endogenous protein kininogen from plasma), have been developed for the treatment of AD. A randomized phase II trial for omiganan demonstrated that topical use of this compound once daily significantly improved inflammatory skin lesions and pruritus in patients with mild-to-moderate AD [23]. DPK-060 has also been studied as a topical ointment for AD patients in a phase I/II trial and has shown a significant decrease in the total microbial colony-forming unit count in eczematous lesions [24].

Furthermore, barrier repair therapies involving the regulation of lipid metabolism are being developed and have shown improvement of the skin barrier in AD subjects [25]. In addition, studies on topical reagents such as BRT-FC-83C, PDI-192, and IDP-124, or external devices such as nocturnal temperature-controlled laminar airflow, with unknown mechanisms but with potential effects on the restoration of the skin barrier, have been completed, although the results have not yet been published [26-30].

Table 1 summarizes the recent barrier repair therapies in AD under clinical trials.

3. Therapy Targeting Type 2 Immunity

Type 2 immunity involves the activity of type 2 helper T (Th2) cells; type 2 innate lymphoid cells (ILC2s); eosinophils; mast cells; basophils; Th2 cytokines such as interleukin (IL)-4, IL-5 and IL-13; and immunoglobulin (Ig) E. Type 2 immunity is thought to play a pivotal role in the development of AD by driving various inflammatory responses and IgE synthesis [1, 9, 31]. Therefore, targeting the downstream components of the Th2 pathway has led to revolutionized treatments for allergic conditions, including AD. Table 2 summarizes ongoing current drugs and respective clinical trials targeting type 2 immunity.

Table 2. Interventional clinical trials with type 2 immunity inhibiting therapies in atopic dermatitis

Target	Treatment	Population/ severity	Phase of current development/status	NCT No.	Route
IL-4Rα	Dupilumab/ Dupixent/ REGN668/ SAR231893	18-65y/MS	IV/active, not recruiting	NCT03389893	SC
		>18y/MS	IV/recruiting	NCT03293030	SC
		>18y/MS	IV/recruiting	NCT03667014	SC
		>18y/MS	IV/recruiting	NCT04033367	SC
		6m-18y/MMS	III/enrolling by invitation	NCT02612454	SC
		6-12y/S	III/completed	NCT03345914	SC
		12-18y/MS	III/completed	NCT03054428	SC
		>18y/MS	III/active, not recruiting	NCT01949311	SC
		>18y/MS	III/completed	NCT03912259	SC
		>18y/S	III/completed	NCT02755649	SC
		>18y/MS	III/completed	NCT02260986	SC
		>18y/MS	III/completed	NCT02277743	SC
		>18y/MS	III/completed	NCT02277769	SC
IL-4/ IL-13	Pitrakinra/ AER 001	>18y/MS	IIa/completed	NCT00676884	SC
IL-13	Tralokinumab	>12y/MS	III/recruiting	NCT03587805	SC
		>18y/S	III/recruiting	NCT03761537	SC
		12-17y/MS	III/active, not recruiting	NCT03526861	SC
		>18y/MS	III/completed	NCT03363854	SC
		>18y/MS	III/completed	NCT03160885	SC
		>18y/MS	III/completed	NCT03131648	SC
	Lebrikizumab	>12y/MS	III/suspended*	NCT04250350	SC
		>12y/MS	III/suspended*	NCT04178967	SC
		>12y/MS	III/suspended*	NCT04146363	SC
		>12y/MS	III/suspended*	NCT04250337	SC
		18-75y/MS	II/completed	NCT02465606	SC
		>18y/MS	IIb/completed	NCT03443024	SC
		18-75y/MS	II/completed	NCT02340234	SC
IL-13Rα1	ASLAN004	>18y/MS	Ib/recruiting	NCT04090229	SC
IL-5R	Benralizumab	18-65y/MS	II/recruiting	NCT03563066	SC
IL-5	Mepolizumab	18-70y/MS	II/terminated*	NCT03055195	SC
TSLP	Tezepelumab/ AMG157/ MEDI9929	18-75y/MS	IIb/recruiting	NCT03809663	SC
		18-75y/MS	IIa/completed	NCT02525094	SC
IL-33	REGN3500/ SAR440340	18-75y/MS	IIa/active, not recruiting	NCT03736967	SC
		18-75y/MS	IIb/active, not recruiting	NCT03738423	SC
	Etokimab/ ANB020	18-75y/MS	II/recruiting	NCT03533751	SC

Table 2. (Continued)

Target	Treatment	Population/ severity	Phase of current development/status	NCT No.	Route
IL-33	MEDI3506	18-75y/MS	II/active, not recruiting	NCT04212169	SC/IV
IL-33R	CNTO 7160	18-55y/MMS	I/completed	NCT02345928	IV
	MSTT1041A	18-75y/MS	II/active, not recruiting	NCT03747575	SC
IgE	XmAb7195	18-50y/MS	I/completed	NCT02148744	IV
	Xolair/ Omalizumab	4-19y/S	IV/completed	NCT02300701	SC
		12-60y/MMS	IV/completed	NCT00822783	SC
	Ligelizumab	18-65y/MS	II/completed	NCT01552629	SC
	MEDI4212	18-60y/MMS	I/completed	NCT01544348	SC/IV
	Immuno-adsorption	18-70y/S	II/unknown	NCT02365246	AP

IL-13Rα1: IL-13 receptor α1 subunit; MM: mild-to-moderate; MS: moderate-to-severe; MMS: mild, moderate and severe; S: severe; IV: intravenous injection; IM: intramuscular injection; SC: subcutaneous injection; AP: apheresis; Suspended*: temporary enrollment suspension to manage patient safety due to coronavirus disease 2019 (COVID-19); Terminated*: study reached pre-determined futility criteria following interim analysis.

3.1. Targeting IL-4 and/or IL-13

IL-4 and IL-13 are the two most important cytokines that contribute to the induction and effector phases of type 2 inflammation and the regulation of IgE synthesis [32]. Dupilumab, a systemic biologic targeting IL-4 receptor α (IL-4Ra), a shared receptor subunit for IL-4 and IL-13, is able to downregulate the markers of epidermal proliferation and inflammatory mediators and to upregulate epidermal barrier proteins and lipid metabolism proteins, resulting in the improvement of affected skin [33]. Dupilumab has been used in a series of clinical trials since 2010 and was approved by the FDA in 2017 for the treatment of patients with moderate-to-severe AD. In two phase III trials involving patients with AD, dupilumab improved both the signs and the symptoms of AD, including pruritus, symptoms of anxiety and depression, and the quality of life, compared with placebo [34]. To study the long-term efficacy and safety of dupilumab plus a TCS in adults with moderate-to-severe AD, a phase III trial involving 740 patients was conducted and showed that, by week 52, more than 60% of patients treated with dupilumab and a TCS weekly or biweekly achieved EASI-75, compared to 22% in the patients treated with placebo [35]. Moreover, rapid improvement in pruritus and flares was reached in AD patients with dupilumab treatment in these trials [36, 37]. Two randomized double-blind, placebo-controlled, phase IV studies evaluating the effect of dupilumab on sleep and the quality of life in moderate-to-severe AD adult patients are ongoing [38-39].

The highest prevalence of AD is found in the pediatric and adolescent populations worldwide [40]. In a 16-week, randomized, placebo-controlled phase III trial involving adolescents with AD from 12 to 18 years old, dupilumab improved AD signs, symptoms, and the quality of life [41]. Moreover, an autoinjector device to deliver dupilumab has been compared to delivery by a prefilled syringe in moderate-to-severe AD patients aged 12 years and older, and the results are awaited [42]. The most common adverse events in most trials are injection-site reactions, skin infections, nasopharyngitis, upper respiratory tract infection, and conjunctivitis [34, 35, 41, 43].

In addition to IL-4Ra, targeting either IL-4 or IL-13 is another emerging therapeutic strategy for AD treatment. Pitrakinra, a dual antagonist for IL-4/IL-13, and tralokinumab and lebrikizumab, humanized monoclonal antibodies that block signaling downstream of IL-13, have been developed to tackle type 2 inflammation. Pitrakinra was studied in patients with moderate-to-severe AD in a phase IIa study; however, no results are available to date [44]. The newest published data of a phase IIb trial for tralokinumab in adults with moderate-to-severe AD showed that 300 mg of tralokinumab significantly improved the change from baseline in EASI score versus placebo at week 12 [45]. Another set of phase III trials to evaluate tralokinumab monotherapy or tralokinumab in combination with a TCS in moderate-to-severe AD adults was completed last year (2019) without available results to date. Moreover, two phase III trials to evaluate tralokinumab monotherapy in adolescent AD patients are ongoing [46, 47]. In addition, two recent randomized, double-blind, placebo-controlled, phase II studies showed that lebrikizumab injection at a dose of 125 mg every 4 weeks significantly improved the EASI score versus placebo at week 12 [48] or week 16 [49]. The most frequent adverse effects induced by tralokinumab were nasopharyngitis, upper respiratory tract infection, headache, and the exacerbation of AD, while lebrikizumab was well tolerated [48, 50].

3.2. Targeting IL-5 and Its Receptor

IL-5 plays a critical role in the recruitment, activation, differentiation, and survival of eosinophils [51, 52]. Therefore, anti-IL-5 antibody is considered a potential therapeutic agent in subjects with AD by reducing the production and survival of eosinophils [53-55]. A multicenter, randomized, double-blind, placebo-controlled, parallel-group phase II clinical trial initiated to address the efficacy and safety of mepolizumab, an anti-IL-5 biologic, confirmed that significantly more patients achieved the Investigator's Global Assessment (IGA) endpoint at week 16 and a marked decrease in blood eosinophil count from baseline at weeks 4, 8, and 16 in the mepolizumab group vs the placebo group [56]. In this study, mepolizumab was generally well tolerated [56]. In addition to mepolizumab, benralizumab, a biologic agent against the α-chain of the IL-5 receptor, was initially developed for the treatment of asthma. A randomized, double-blind, parallel group, placebo-controlled phase II study is being conducted to investigate the effect of benralizumab on the regulation of eosinophils, basophils and ILC2s in adult patients with moderate-to-severe AD [57].

3.3. Targeting IL-33 and Its Receptor

IL-33, an alarmin cytokine, has been found to be involved in the complex pathogenesis of AD since the past decade [58]. IL-33 is constitutively expressed in epithelial cells and is rapidly released in response to damage and stress conditions such as infection, injury, and inflammation [59]. By binding to its heterodimeric receptor composed of suppressor of tumorigenicity-2 (ST2) and IL-1 receptor accessory protein

(IL-1RAcP), IL-33 stimulates Th2-polarized $CD4^+$ T cells [60], triggers mast cell degranulation [61], and induces a large amount of IL-4 production from basophils [60] and Th2 cytokines, including IL-5 and IL-13, from ILC2s [62]. Phase I and II trials involving patients with AD have been initiated for etokimab and REGN3500, which target IL-33, and CNTO 7160, an anti-ST2 receptor monoclonal antibody. To date, among these trials, one proof-of-concept trial of etokimab showed that single systemic administration of etokimab led to rapid and sustained clinical effects, with a reduction in peripheral eosinophils at day 29 in moderate-to-severe AD adult patients [63]. Etokimab was generally well tolerated in this study, and the most common adverse events included infections and infestations, headache, upper respiratory tract infection, urinary tract infection and peripheral swelling [63]. Moreover, CNTO 7160 was well tolerated in healthy subjects and AD patients in a first-in-human study but did not show apparent clinical improvements [64].

3.4. Targeting Thymic Stromal Lymphopoietin (TSLP) and Its Receptor

TSLP, an IL-2 family cytokine produced by skin keratinocytes and epithelial cells in the lung and gut in response to damage, is pivotal to allergic diseases mediated by the Th2 response, including AD [65-67]. The TSLP/TSLP receptor (TSLPR) axis regulates barrier immunity by driving the activation of immature dendritic cells, mast cells, basophils, eosinophils and lymphocytes into a type 2 polarizing phenotype [67-69]. Tezepelumab, a human monoclonal antibody blocking TSLP, has been designed for the treatment of asthma and AD [70]. In a phase IIa study, 113 patients were randomized 1:1 to receive 280 mg tezepelumab subcutaneously or placebo every 2 weeks, plus a TCS. A numerically greater percentage of tezepelumab-plus-TCS-treated patients achieved EASI50 than placebo-plus-TCS-treated patients [71]. Treatment-emergent adverse events, including injection-site erythema, were similar between treatment groups [71]. In addition, ASP7266, a novel recombinant human

IgG1 monoclonal antibody targeting TSLPR, has been developed for the treatment of allergen-induced inflammation [72]. However, more data are needed to test its therapeutic effect and safety in patients with AD.

3.5. Targeting IgE

IgE mediates hypersensitivity reactions responsible for most atopic diseases, including AD. Although an anti-IgE biologic, omalizumab, has been shown to be effective in a subgroup of asthma patients [73], the results of this compound to treat adult patients with AD are controversial [74]. However, recently, the largest phase IV trial for omalizumab showed that this drug significantly reduced the severity of AD and improved the quality of life in a pediatric population with severe AD despite highly elevated total IgE levels at baseline [75, 76]. A study targeting IgE with a combination of omalizumab and immunoglobulin apheresis also suggested that severe AD patients could obtain improvement following this treatment [77]. Another anti-IgE therapy, MEDI4212, showed rapid suppression of free serum IgE from AD patients with elevated IgE levels to a greater extent than omalizumab and was well tolerated by the patients [78]. Another anti-IgE biologic, ligelizumab, has completed few clinical trials, but no results are available to date [79, 80]. Further studies are needed to evaluate whether the strategy targeting IgE is more promising for some subsets of AD, particularly in the pediatric population.

4. Inhibiting the Activation of Other Helper T Cell Pathways

In addition to the Th2 pathway, other helper T cell pathways, such as the Th17 (IL-17A, IL-17C)/IL-23 [81-83] and Th22 (IL-22) [84-86] pathways, have also been involved in the pathogenesis of AD. Recently, multiple therapeutic strategies targeting these pathways have been conducted for AD treatment (Table 3). Secukinumab, a fully human anti-

IL-17A monoclonal antibody, was reported to successfully improve AD with remarkable clinical, histological, and molecular responses in an Asian patient with severe AD [87]. However, a recent phase II study of the treatment of moderate-to-severe AD with secukinumab showed neither significant clinical nor molecular improvement, even for high Th17-skewing subtypes [88]. Another phase II study for secukinumab is being conducted to confirm the above results [89]. IL-17C exacerbates epithelial inflammation in patients with AD [90], and the neutralization of IL-17C with MOR106 reduces skin inflammation in an AD mouse model [91]. Although a phase I study for the assessment of safety, tolerability and pharmacokinetics of multiple ascending doses of MOR106 in moderate-to-severe AD subjects has been completed, the clinical development for this compound in AD has been stopped due its ineffectiveness demonstrated in two of the newest phase II trials [92, 93]. Although ustekinumab, an anti-IL-12/23 monoclonal antibody, has been licensed for the treatment of moderate-to-severe psoriasis [94], some case reports have shown controversial results regarding ustekinumab in AD patients.

Table 3. Interventional clinical trials with other helper T-cell pathways targeting therapies in atopic dermatitis

Target	Treatment	Population/ severity	Phase of current development/status	NCT No.	Route
IL-17A	Secukinumab/ Cosentyx	>18y/MS	II/completed	NCT02594098	SC
		18-85y/MS	II/active, not recruiting	NCT03568136	SC
IL-17C	MOR106/ ZPL389	18-65y/MS	II/stopped	NCT03568071	IV
		18-65y/MS	II/stopped	NCT03864627	IV
		18-65y/MS	I/completed	NCT02739009	IV
IL-12/23	Ustekinumab	18-75/MS	II/completed	NCT01806662	SC
		20-65/S	II/completed	NCT01945086	SC
IL-23	Risankizumab	>12y/MS	II/recruiting	NCT03706040	SC
IL-22	Fezakinumab/ ILV-094	18-75y/MS	II/completed	NCT01941537	IV
	ARGX 112/ LEO 138559	18-55y/ MMS	I/suspended*	NCT03514511	SC/IV

MS: moderate-to-severe; MMS: mild, moderate and severe; S: severe; IV: intravenous injection; SC: subcutaneous injection.

Furthermore, a recent well-conducted small phase II study has shown that 45 mg and 90 mg ustekinumab did not demonstrate significant efficacy in 79 Japanese patients with severe AD [95].

IL-22 blockade with fezakinumab is another emerging targeted strategy for AD treatment. A recent randomized, double-blind, phase IIa trial described that in the severe AD subset, the decline in IGA was significantly higher in fezakinumab-treated patients than in placebo-treated patients [96], and significant downregulation of multiple immune pathways, including Th1/CXCL9, Th2/CCL18/CCL22, Th17/CCL20/ DEFB4A, and Th22/IL-22/S100As, was observed only in the high-dose IL-22 drug group [97]. Common adverse events in this study involved upper respiratory tract infections [96].

5. Broad-Targeting Therapy

The pathogenesis of AD involves various immune pathways that are interconnected. Therefore, the inhibition of several immune pathways by broad-targeting agents might be a potent strategy for all subsets of AD patients. Broad-targeting therapeutics being developed for AD treatment are summarized in Table 4.

Table 4. Interventional clinical trials with broad-targeting therapies in atopic dermatitis

Target	Treatment	Population/ severity	Phase of current development/status	NCT No.	Route
JAK1	Abrocitinib/ PF-04965842	>18y/MS	IIIb/not yet recruiting	NCT04345367	Oral
		12-17y/MS	III/recruiting	NCT03796676	Oral
		>12y/MS	III/active, not recruiting	NCT03627767	Oral
		>12y/MS	III/enrolling by invitation	NCT03422822	Oral
		>18y/MS	III/completed	NCT03720470	Oral
		>12y/MS	III/completed	NCT03575871	Oral
		>12y/MS	III/completed	NCT03349060	Oral

Target	Treatment	Population/ severity	Phase of current development/status	NCT No.	Route
JAK1	Upadacitinib/ ABT-494/ RINVOQ	18-75y/MS	IIIb/recruiting	NCT03738397	Oral
		18-75y/MS	IIIb/recruiting	NCT04195698	Oral
		12-75y/MS	III/recruiting	NCT03569293	Oral
		12-75y/MS	III/recruiting	NCT03568318	Oral
		12-75y/MS	III/recruiting	NCT03607422	Oral
		12-75y/MS	III/active, not recruiting	NCT03661138	Oral
	SHR0302	18-75y/MS	II/recruiting	NCT04162899	Oral
JAK 1/2	Baricitinib/ LY3009104	>18y/MS	III/enrolling by invitation	NCT03559270	Oral
		2-17y/MS	III/recruiting	NCT03952559	Oral
		>18y/MS	III/active, not recruiting	NCT03435081	Oral
		>18y/MS	III/active, not recruiting	NCT03334435	Oral
		>18y/MS	III/Active, not recruiting	NCT03428100	Oral
		>18y/MS	III/completed	NCT03334422	Oral
		>18y/MS	III/completed	NCT03334396	Oral
		>18y/MS	III/completed	NCT03733301	Oral
	Ruxolitinib/ INCB018424	>12y/Mo	III/active, not recruiting	NCT03745651	Topical
		>12y/Mo	III/active, not recruiting	NCT03745638	Topical
		18-70y/Mo	II/completed	NCT03011892	Topical
JAK 1/3	ATI-502	>18y/MS	II/completed	NCT03585296	Topical
JAK1/ 2/3/ TRK2	Tofacitinib	18-60y/MM	IIa/completed	NCT02001181	Topical
	PF-06700841	12-75y/MM	IIb/recruiting	NCT03903822	Topical
	Delgocitinib	>18y/MMS	IIb/active, not recruiting	NCT03725722	Topical
		>2y/MS	I/recruiting	NCT03826901	Topical
JAK/ SYK	ASN002	18-75y/MS	II/enrolling by invitation	NCT03654755	Oral
		18-75y/MS	IIb/completed	NCT03531957	Oral
H4R	ZPL-893787/ ZPL-389	18-65y/MS	II/completed	NCT02424253	Oral
		>18y/MMS	II/recruiting	NCT03948334	Oral
	JNJ-39758979	20-65y/Mo	II/terminated	NCT01497119	Oral
PDE4	Apremilast/ Otezla/ CC-10004	>18y/MS	II/not yet recruiting	NCT04306965	Oral
		18-85y/MS	II/recruiting	NCT03160248	Oral
		>18y/MS	II/completed	NCT02087943	Oral
		>18y/MS	II/completed	NCT01393158	Oral
		>18y/MS	II/completed	NCT00931242	Oral
	KHK4577	20-65y/MS	II/completed	NCT02004119	Oral
	Difamilast/ OPA-15406/ MM36	>2y/MMS	II/recruiting	NCT03961529	Topical
		2-14y/MS	III/completed	NCT03911401	Topical
		15-70y/MS	III/completed	NCT03908970	Topical

Table 4. (Continued)

Target	Treatment	Population/ severity	Phase of current development/status	NCT No.	Route
PDE4	Lotamilast/ RVT-501/ E6005	12-70y/MM	II/completed	NCT02950922	Topical
		2-17y/MM	II/completed	NCT03394677	Topical
		20-65y/MMS	II/completed	NCT01461941	Topical
		2-15y/MMS	I/II/completed	NCT02094235	Topical
	AN2728/ PF-06930164	>18y/MM	IV/recruiting	NCT03868098	Topical
		3-24m/MM	IV/completed	NCT03356977	Topical
		>2y/MM	IIIb/IV/completed	NCT03539601	Topical
	DRM02	18-70y/Mi	II/completed	NCT01993420	Topical
	Roflumilast/ ARQ-151/ GW842470X	18-65y/Mo	IIa/completed	NCT01856764	Topical
		>12y/MM	II/completed	NCT03916081	Topical
		18-65y/Mo	II/completed	NCT00354510	Topical
	LEO 29102	18-65y/MM	II/completed	NCT01447758	Topical
	LEO 32731	>18y/MM	I/completed	NCT02496546	Topical
	LEO 39652	>18y/MM	I/completed	NCT02219633	Topical
OX40	KHK4083	>18y/MS	II/not yet recruiting	NCT03703102	SC
		>20y/MS	I/completed	NCT03096223	SC
	ISB 830/ GBR 830	>18y/MS	IIb/recruiting	NCT03568162	SC
		>18y/MS	II/completed	NCT02683928	SC
OX40L	KY1005	18-75y/MS	II/not yet recruiting	NCT03754309	SC/IV
AhR	Tapinarof/ GSK2894512/ Benvitimod/ WBI 1001	12-65y/MS	II/completed	NCT02564055	Topical
		18-65y/MM	IIb/completed	NCT01098734	Topical
CRTH2-R	Fevipiprant/ QAW039	18-65y/MS	II/completed	NCT01785602	Oral
	OC000459/ Timapiprant	18-48y/MS	II/completed	NCT02002208	Oral
	KHK4577	20-64y/MS	II/completed	NCT02004119	Oral
IL-1	Anakinra	10-30y/S	I/terminated	NCT01122914	IV
CCR4	RPT193	18-65y/MS	Ib/recruiting	NCT04271514	Oral
TLR/ GPCR	DMT210	>12y/MM	II/completed	NCT02949960	Topical
CD11a	Efalizumab	>18y/MS	II/completed	NCT00146003	SC
CD200R	LY 3454738	18-65y/MMS	I/suspended*	NCT03750643	IV
ORAI1	DS-2741a	>20y/MMS	I/recruiting	NCT04211415	SC
Treg	NKTR-358/ LY3471851	18-70y/MMS	I/suspended	NCT04081350	SC
5-HT	AM1030	18-65y/MMS	I/II/completed	NCT02379910	Topical
5-LO	Q301/ zileuton	12-70y/MM	II/completed	NCT03571620	Topical
		>18y/MS	II/completed	NCT02426359	Topical
SHIP-1	AQX-1125	18-65y/MM	II/completed	NCT02324972	Oral
cPLA2	PF 5212372	18-65y/MS	I/II/completed	NCT02795832	Topical

Target	Treatment	Population/ severity	Phase of current development/status	NCT No.	Route
S1P1R	Etrasimod	18-70y/MS	II/recruiting	NCT04162769	Oral
CB1R	BTX-1204	12-70y/Mo	II/completed	NCT03824405	Topical
LFA-3	Alefacept	>18y/MS	IV/completed	NCT00832585	IM

S1P1R: sphingosine-1-phosphate-1; CB1R: cannabinoid receptor type 1 receptor; Treg: regulatory T cell; 5-HT:5-hydroxytryptamine; 5-LO: 5-lipoxygenase; cPLA2: cytosolic phospholipase A2; LFA-3: leukocyte function antigen-3; MM: mild-to-moderate; MS: moderate-to-severe; MMS: mild, moderate and severe; Mi: mild; Mo: moderate; S: severe; IV: intravenous injection; IM: intramuscular injection; SC: subcutaneous injection; Suspended*: temporary enrollment suspension to manage patient safety due to COVID-19.

5.1. Targeting TNF-α

Although the two anti-TNF-α antibodies, infliximab [98] and etanercept [99], have failed in the treatment of patients with AD, the inhibition of the TNF receptor (OX40) by GBR-830 was shown to induce significant clinical changes in adult patients with moderate-to-severe AD [100]. A new phase IIb clinical trial using GBR-830 is being initiated [101]. Furthermore, other anti-OX40 agents, such as KHK4083 and KY1005, are being evaluated in phase II studies involving patients with AD [102, 103].

5.2. Targeting the Aryl Hydrocarbon Receptor

The aryl hydrocarbon receptor (AhR), a ubiquitously expressed ligand-activated transcription factor, is a chemical sensor expressed on skin cells, including keratinocytes, sebocytes, fibroblasts, dendritic cells, and other immune cells [104]. The AhR has gained increased attention owing to its ability to modulate the oxidative and antioxidative balance, epidermal differentiation and inflammation in the skin [105, 106]. Notably, several randomized phase II studies have reported that topical application of the natural AhR agonist tapinarof is efficacious and well-tolerated in adult patients with AD [107-110].

5.3. Targeting Phosphodiesterase 4 (PDE4)

PDE4 is a key regulator of inflammatory cytokine production. This enzyme converts cyclic adenosine monophosphate (cAMP) into the 50-AMP molecule, which modulates the generation of proinflammatory (increased PDE4) or anti-inflammatory (decreased PDE4) cytokines by immune cells [111]. PDE4 activity is increased in patients with AD, and this enzyme has been targeted in AD treatment by increasing intracellular cAMP and reducing the production of inflammatory cytokines [112, 113]. PDE4 inhibitors, including crisaborole, E6005, MM36, DRM02, roflumilast and LEO 29102, are currently under development. Among them, topical boron-based crisaborole cream was approved in 2016 by the FDA for children and adult patients with mild-to-moderate AD [114]. In two pivotal phase III studies, crisaborole-treated patients achieved improved IGA score and improvements in pruritus compared with vehicle-treated patients [114]. A number of trials also showed that clinical improvement could be achieved in children and adults with mild-to-moderate AD with other topical PDE4 inhibitors, such as E6005 [115-117], OPA-15406 [118-120] and LEO29102 [121]. The adverse effects included mild-to-moderate worsening of AD, application-site reactions, and vulvovaginal yeast infections [115-120]. DRM-02, a topical gel under study in rosacea and psoriasis, has also completed a phase II trial in AD patients; however, the results are not yet available [121].

5.4. Janus Kinase (JAK) Inhibitors

The JAK family consists of JAK1, JAK2, JAK3 and tyrosine kinase 2 (TYK2), which, together with the signal transducer and activator of transcription (STAT) family, are involved in the signaling of polar cytokines such as Th2 (IL-4, IL-5, IL-13, IL-33, TSLP), Th17 (IL-17A)/IL-23, and Th22 (IL-22) that contribute to AD pathogenesis [122, 123]. Therefore, JAK inhibitors are promising targets for AD treatment.

Tofacitinib, a pan-JAK antagonist, was topically applied in a phase IIa placebo-controlled clinical trial of 69 adult patients with mild-to-moderate AD, and the percentage change from baseline in the EASI score was significantly decreased without serious adverse events in those receiving tofacitinib compared with those receiving placebo [124]. Furthermore, a systemic administration of tofacitinib in a small open-label clinical trial in six moderate-to-severe AD patients showed a decrease in SCORAD with no serious adverse events noted [125].

Another pan-JAK inhibitor, delgocitinib, was tested in two phase I studies and showed that both 1% and 3% delgocitinib ointments were efficacious in reducing AD severity and pruritus [126]. Moreover, in a phase II vehicle-controlled clinical study, 327 Japanese adult patients with moderate-to-severe AD achieved significant improvement in EASI score, modified EASI score and IGA score by following treatment with delgocitinib ointment (0.25%, 0.5%, 1%, or 3%) compared with vehicle ointment [127].

Baricitinib, an oral selective JAK 1/2 antagonist, effectively improved AD in a phase II study with concomitant use of a TCS [128], allowing this biologic to advance into phase III trials for baricitinib monotherapy versus placebo in moderate-to-severe AD. In two of these phase III monotherapy trials, adults with moderate-to-severe AD randomly received baricitinib once daily for 16 weeks, and significant improvement of clinical signs and symptoms could be observed with 2 mg and 4 mg baricitinib compared with placebo [129]. Baricitinib was mostly well-tolerated, but there were adverse events such as headache, nasopharyngitis and increased blood creatine phosphokinase [130]. Another topical selective JAK 1/2 inhibitor, ruxolitinib, showed significant improvements in an itch numerical rating scale in a randomized phase II trial involving 307 adult AD patients, with only mild or moderate adverse events [131, 132]. Currently, two phase III studies and a phase I open-label study are being conducted using ruxolitinib cream in adolescent and pediatric AD patients [133-135].

Abrocitinib, upadacitinib and SHR0302 are oral selective JAK1 inhibitors. A randomized, double-blinded, placebo-controlled phase IIb trial reported that 44.5% of AD patients treated with abrocitinib versus

6.3% of patients treated with a placebo showed clinical improvement as assessed by IGA score [136]. Additionally, the newest phase III clinical trial showed that monotherapy with oral abrocitinib was effective and well tolerated in adolescents and adults with moderate-to-severe AD [137]. Concerning upadacitinib, it showed impressive clinical outcomes in a phase IIb trial. Upadacitinib is generally well tolerated, with adverse effects such as upper respiratory tract infection, AD worsening, and acne [138]. Currently, multiple phase III clinical trials are being evaluated for the efficacy and safety of upadacitinib in adult and adolescent AD. A proof-of-concept trial is analyzing the use of SHR0302 in adult patients with moderate-to-severe AD [139]. These trials will help define the efficacy and safety of JAK inhibitors in AD patients. Although JAK inhibitors have promising effects for AD treatment, long-term safety is yet to be determined because the safety profiles differ among different agents.

5.5. Histamine Receptor Type 4 Antagonists

The histamine receptor type 4 (H4R), which is expressed on keratinocytes and immune cells, plays a key role in pruritus and Th2- and Th17-mediated inflammation [140, 141]. Therefore, H4R antagonists are thought to be another class of broad-acting agents for AD [142]. Unlike H1R inhibitors used as antipruritic agents, yet mainly as sedative agents in AD, an H4R antagonist, ZPL-389, showed promising improvements in inflammatory skin lesions as assessed by the EASI score in a phase II study [1, 4, 143]. This result raises the question of whether this compound plays primarily an anti-inflammatory role or an antipruritic role in AD. Currently, a long-term study is recruiting to evaluate the safety and efficacy of oral ZPL-389 with concomitant use of a TCS [144].

5.6. Other Broad-Targeting Inhibitors

DMT210 (formerly known as Sig990) is a topical inhibitor expected to disrupt signal transduction by modulating Toll-like receptor and G protein-coupled receptor signaling, leading to the downregulation of proinflammatory cytokines [145]. Furthermore, AM1030 is a topical inhibitor that targets the neurotransmitter serotonin [146]. Both DMT210 and AM1030 have shown anti-inflammatory effects in preclinical studies for the treatment of AD and rosacea by reducing both T cell-dependent and T cell-independent inflammatory responses [145, 146]. These two inhibitors have also been studied in phase II clinical trials for their efficacy in suppressing inflammation and itching in adolescent and adult AD patients [147, 148]. In addition, several other topical agents, including Q301 [149, 150], LEO32731 [151] and LEO39652 [152, 153], are also currently being developed for the treatment of AD. Although the clear mechanism of these formulations is unknown, it is suggested that their anti-inflammatory properties are due to the inhibition of multiple cytokines.

6. Antipruritic Agents

Chronic pruritus is one of the most debilitating and burdensome symptoms of AD [1, 4]. The sensation of pruritus is known to be induced by a variety of histamine-dependent and independent pruritogens, such as IL-31, TSLP, proteases and endothelin-1, through afferent fibers from the skin to the spine and brain, and it is mediated by different neurological mediators, including substance P [154-156]. Therefore, several antipruritic medications are currently being assessed in clinical trials for the treatment of AD (Table 5). Nemolizumab, an anti-IL-31 receptor antibody, is one of the most promising agents to inhibit atopic itch. In a 24-week, randomized, double-blind, multicenter phase II study, subcutaneous injections of nemolizumab significantly improved EASI, IGA, and/or numeric rating scale (NRS)-itch scores in patients with AD, with the dose of 30 mg being the most effective [157]. In another long-term phase IIb study with nemolizumab, it was shown that significant improvement from baseline in pruritus visual analog scale score was maintained/increased from weeks 12 to 64 [158]. The treatment-related adverse events in the above two studies were mild to moderate [157, 158]. Currently, phase II and III studies for nemolizumab are ongoing in adolescent and adult AD patients [159-162].

Table 5. Interventional clinical trials with antipruritic agents in atopic dermatitis

Target	Treatment	Population/ severity	Phases of current development/ status	NCT No.	Route
IL-31	BMS-981164	18-65y/MS	I/completed	NCT01614756	SC/IV
IL-31RA	Nemolizumab/ CIM331	>12y/MS	III/recruiting	NCT03989206	SC
		>12y/MS	III/recruiting	NCT03985943	SC
		>12y/MS	III/recruiting	NCT03989349	SC
		12-17y/MS	II/recruiting	NCT03921411	SC
		>18y/MS	II/completed	NCT03100344	SC
		18-65y/MS	II/completed	NCT01986933	SC
NK1-R	Tradipitant/ VLY-686	18-70y/MMS	II/recruiting	NCT04140695	Oral
		18-70y/MMS	II/completed	NCT03568331	Oral
	Serlopitant/ VPD-737	>18y/MMS	III/active, not recruiting	NCT03540160	Oral
		>13/MMS	II/completed	NCT02975206	Oral
NK1/ NK2R	DNK333	18-60y/MMS	II/completed	NCT01033097	Oral
Opioid	SRD174	>18y/MS	II/completed	NCT00838708	Topical
Opioid receptor	Naltrexone	18-70y/MMS	II/not yet recruiting	NCT04154033	Topical
		18-70y/MMS	II/not yet recruiting	NCT04325802	Topical
κ-Opioid receptor	Asimadoline/ EMD-61753	>18y/MMS	II/completed	NCT02475447	Oral
	Difelikefalin	18-80y/MS	II/recruiting	NCT04018027	Oral
TrkA	CT327	>12y/MM	II/completed	NCT01808157	Topical
TRPV1	PAC-14028	12-70y/MM	III/completed	NCT02965118	Topical
DP-1 receptor	TS-022	18-65y/MS	II/completed	NCT00914186	Topical
Kallikrein -related peptidase	LM 030/ BPR 277	18-65y/MS	I/completed	NCT01428297	Topical

MS: moderate-to-severe; MMS: mild, moderate and severe; IV: intravenous injection; SC: subcutaneous injection.

7. Regulation of the Skin Microbiome

Dysbiosis in the skin microbiome and the deficiency of AMPs enable *Staphylococcus aureus* (*S. aureus*) colonization, leading to inflammation in AD [163]. Consequently, the regulation of microbial diversity and the reduction of *S. aureus* infection have gained focus as nonantibiotic approaches for the treatment of AD. Lysates from a commensal nonpathogenic *Vitreoscilla filiformis* have been developed as a cream for AD in an early prospective, randomized, double-blind, placebo-controlled trial, and SCORAD levels, pruritus, and *S. aureus* colonization were significantly reduced [164]. Recently, the transplantation of commensal strains of coagulase-negative *Staphylococcus*, including *Staphylococcus epidermidis* and *Staphylococcus hominis*, collected from the skin of healthy volunteers but not patients with AD, showed protective function for the skin barrier and the inhibition of *S. aureus* colonization in patients with AD [165]. In addition, topical treatment with another commensal Gram-negative skin bacterium, *Roseomonas mucosa,* also significantly decreased both objective disease measurements and subjective pruritus in patients with AD without causing any adverse events [166]. The only study evaluating whole-skin microbiome transplant by a targeted microbiome transplant lotion containing coagulase-negative *Staphylococcus* as a potential treatment for AD was completed; however, the results have not yet been reported [167].

Anti-staphylococcal therapy specifically targeting *S. aureus* is another novel strategy for regulating the diversity of skin microbes. Staphefekt is an engineered bacteriophage endolysin that selectively kills *S. aureus* without harming skin commensals. Topical use of Staphefekt has successfully treated 3 cases of chronic *S. aureus*-related dermatoses, including eczema [168]. More importantly, no bacterial resistance was found following the use of endolysins, making Staphefekt a promising alternative to traditional antibiotics in reducing the burden of *S. aureus* [169]. A multicenter, placebo-controlled, double-blinded, randomized trial involving 100 moderate-to-severe AD adult participants with topical use of Staphefekt was completed, but no available results to date have been reported [170]. Table 6 summarizes the current skin microbiome-regulated therapies in AD under clinical trials.

Table 6. Interventional clinical trials with skin microbiome-regulated therapies in atopic dermatitis

Treatment	Population/ severity	Phase of current development/status	NCT No.	Route
Staphefekt	>18y/MS	NA/completed	NCT02840955	Topical
Autologous Microbiome Transplant	18-80y/MMS	I/active, not recruiting	NCT01959113	Topical
	18-80y/MMS	I/active, not recruiting	NCT01960764	Topical
	18-80y/MMS	II/active, not recruiting	NCT02144142	Topical
	18-60y/MMS	I/completed	NCT03158012	Topical
TMT	18-60y/MS	I/II/completed	NCT03151148	Topical
V. filiformis	6-70y/S	NA/completed	NCT00509535	Topical
R. mucosa	3-99y/MMS	I/II/completed	NCT03018275	Topical
L. reeuteri	1-8y/MM	NA/recruiting	NCT04265716	Topical
J. lividum	>18y/Mo	II/recruiting	NCT04192513	Topical
FMT	>18y/MS	I/not yet recruiting	NCT04283968	Topical
Maternal microbiota	<15min/H	NA/recruiting	NCT03928431	Topical
Antimicrobial therapeutic clothing	<80y/MS	NA/recruiting	NCT04297215	External device

MM: mild-to-moderate; MS: moderate-to-severe; MMS: mild, moderate and severe; S: severe; H: healthy; TMT: targeted microbiome transplant; FMT: fecal microbial transplantation; *V. filiformis*: *Vitreoscilla filiformis*; *R. mucosa*: *Roseomonas mucosa*; *L. reeuteri*: *Lactobacillus reuteri*; *J. lividum*: *Janthinobacterium lividum*.

Conclusion and Future Considerations

Several novel targeted therapeutic strategies have been exploited following breakthroughs in the understanding of the underlying mechanisms of AD pathogenesis in recent decades. These novel therapeutics with either topical applications or systemic applications serve as a patch, particularly for refractory AD inadequately controlled by TCSs or TCIs. Among these novel therapeutic agents, dupilumab and crisaborole are already available for clinical use. However, most of the novel targeted therapeutic agents may not be available for the treatment of AD in real life because of poor efficacy, a lack of safety data, expensive costs or a lack of enough studies. Therefore, further studies in the translational research of the targeted agents are needed and may help to make more therapeutics amenable for AD treatment in the next decade.

Conflict of Interest

The authors declare no conflicts of interest.

Acknowledgments

The authors wish to thank Michiyo Matsumoto for secretarial assistance. This project was funded in part by a Grant-in-Aid for Scientific Research from the Ministry of Education, Culture, Sports, Science and Technology, Japan (Grant Number: 26461703 to F.N.).

References

[1] Brunello, L. (2018). Atopic dermatitis. *Nat Rev Dis Primers*, 4(1):2.

[2] Cheng, R., Zhang, H., Zong, W., Tang, J., Han, X., Zhang, L., Zhang, X., Gu, H., Shu, Y., Peng, G., Huang, L., Liu, Q., Gao, X., Guo, Y., and Yao, Z. (2020). Development and validation of new diagnostic criteria for atopic dermatitis in children of China. *J Eur Acad Dermatol Venereol*, 34(3):542-548.

[3] Tsai, T. F., Rajagopalan, M., Chu, C. Y., Encarnacion, L., Gerber, R. A., Santos-Estrella, P., Llamado, L., and Tallman, A. M. (2019). Burden of atopic dermatitis in Asia. *J Dermatol*, 46(10), 825-834.

[4] Katoh, N., Ohya, Y., Ikeda, M., Ebihara, T., Katayama, I., Saeki, H., Shimojo, N., Tanaka, A., Nakahara, T., Nagao, M., Hide, M., Fujita, Y., Fujisawa, T., Futamura, M., Masuda, K., Murota, H., Yamamoto-

Hanada, K., and Committee for Clinical Practice Guidelines for the Management of Atopic Dermatitis 2018, Japanasese Society of Allergology, Japanese Dermatology Association (2020). Japanese guidelines for atopic dermatitis 2020. *Allergol Int*. pii: S1323-8930(20)30018-6.

[5] Atherton, D. J. (2003). Topical corticosteroids in atopic dermatitis. *BMJ*, 327(7421):942-943.

[6] Roekevisch, E., Spuls, P. I., Kuester, D., Limpens, J., and Schmitt, J. (2014). Efficacy and safety of systemic treatments for moderate-to-severe atopic dermatitis: a systematic review. *J Allergy Clin Immunol*, 133(2):429-438.

[7] Ashcroft, D. M., Dimmock, P., Garside, R., Stein, K., and Williams, H. C. (2005). Efficacy and tolerability of topical pimecrolimus and tacrolimus in the treatment of atopic dermatitis: meta-analysis of randomised controlled trials. *BMJ*, 330(7490):516.

[8] Aaronson, D. W. (2006). The "black box" warning and allergy drugs. *J Allergy Clin Immunol*, 117(1):40-44.

[9] Elias, P. M., and Steinhoff, M. (2008). "Outside-to-inside" (and now back to "outside") pathogenic mechanisms in atopic dermatitis. *J Invest Dermatol*, 128(5):1067-1070.

[10] Werfel, T., Allam, J. P., Biedermann, T., Eyerich, K., Gilles, S., Guttman-Yassky, E., Hoetzenecker, W., Knol, E., Simon, H. U., Wollenberg, A., Bieber, T., Lauener, R., Schmid-Grendelmeier, P., Traidl-Hoffmann, C., and Akdis, C. A. (2016). Cellular and molecular immunologic mechanisms in patients with atopic dermatitis. *J Allergy Clin Immunol*, 138(2):336-349.

[11] Dhand, A., and Aminoff, M. J. (2014). The neurology of itch. *Brain*, 137(Pt 2):313-322.

[12] Rachana, A., and Judith, A. W. (2014). Skin barrier defects in atopic dermatitis. *Curr Allergy Asthma Rep*, 14(5):433.

[13] Hatano, Y., Man, M. Q., Uchida, Y., Crumrine, D., Mauro, T. M., Feingold, K. R., Elias, P. M., and Holleran, W. M. (2010). Murine atopic dermatitis responds to peroxisome proliferator-activated

receptors alpha and beta/delta (but not gamma) and liver X receptor activators. *J Allergy Clin Immunol*, 125(1):160-169.

[14] Czarnowicki, T., Dohlman, A. B., Malik, K., Antonini, D., Bissonnette, R., Chan, T. C., Zhou, L., Wen, H. C., Estrada, Y., Xu, H., Bryson, C., Shen, J., Lala, D., Ma'ayan, A., McGeehan, G., Gregg, R., and Guttman-Yassky, E. (2018). Effect of short-term liver X receptor activation on epidermal barrier features in mild to moderate atopic dermatitis: A randomized controlled trial. *Ann Allergy Asthma Immunol*, 120(6):631-640.

[15] Hoste, E., Kemperman, P., Devos, M., Denecker, G., Kezic, S., Yau, N., Gilbert, B., Lippens, S., De Groote, P., Roelandt, R., Van Damme, P., Gevaert, K., Presland, R. B., Takahara, H., Puppels, G., Caspers, P., Vandenabeele, P., and Declercq, W. (2011). Caspase-14 is required for filaggrin degradation to natural moisturizing factors in the skin. *J Invest Dermatol*, 131(11):2233-2241.

[16] Kezic, S., Kemperman, P. M., Koster, E. S., de Jongh, C. M., Thio, H. B., Campbell, L. E., Irvine, A. D., McLean, W. H., Puppels, G. J., and Caspers, P. J. (2008). Loss-offunction mutations in the filaggrin gene lead to reduced level of natural moisturizing factor in the stratum corneum. *J Invest Dermatol*, 128(8):2117-2119.

[17] Kezic, S., O'Regan, G. M., Yau, N., Sandilands, A., Chen, H., Campbell, L. E., Kroboth, K., Watson, R., Rowland, M., McLean, W. H., and Irvine, A. D. (2011). Levels of filaggrin degradation products are influenced by both filaggrin genotype and atopic dermatitis severity. *Allergy*, 66(7):934-940.

[18] O'Regan, G. M., Kemperman, P. M., Sandilands, A., Chen, H., Campbell, L. E., Kroboth, K., Watson, R., Rowland, M., Puppels, G. J., McLean, W. H., Caspers, P. J., and Irvine, A. D. (2010). Raman profiles of the stratum corneum define 3 filaggrin genotype-determined atopic dermatitis endophenotypes. *J Allergy Clin Immunol*, 126(3):574-580.

[19] Peltonen, J. M., Pylkkänen, L., Jansén, C. T., Volanen, I., Lehtinen, T., Laihia, J. K., and Leino, L. (2014). Three randomised phase I/IIa trials of 5% cis-urocanic acid emulsion cream in healthy adult

subjects and in patients with atopic dermatitis. *Acta Derm Venereol*, 94(4):415-420.

[20] Niyonsaba, F., Kiatsurayanon, C., Chieosilapatham, P., and Ogawa, H. (2017). Friends or foes? Host defense (antimicrobial) peptides and proteins in human skin diseases. *Exp Dermatol*, 26(11):989-998.

[21] Chieosilapatham, P., Ikeda, S., Ogawa, H., and Niyonsaba, F. (2018). Tissue-specific regulation of innate immune responses by human cathelicidin LL-37. *Curr Pharm Des*, 24(10):1079-1091.

[22] Kiatsurayanon, C., Ogawa, H., and Niyonsaba, F. (2018). The role of host defense peptide human β-defensins in the maintenance of skin barriers. *Curr Pharm Des*, 24(10):1092-1099.

[23] Niemeyer-van der Kolk, T., van der Wall, H., Hogendoorn, G. K., Rijneveld, R., Luijten, S., van Alewijk, D., van den Munckhof, E., de Kam, M. L., Feiss, G. L., Prens, E. P., Burggraaf, J., Rissmann, R., and van Doorn, M. (2020). Pharmacodynamic effects of topical omiganan in patients with mild to moderate atopic dermatitis in a randomized, placebo-controlled, phase II trial. *Clin Transl Sci*. Accessed June 22, 2020. doi: 10.1111/cts.12792.

[24] Margit, M., *Identifier NCT01522391. A randomized, double-blinded placebo-controlled study to investigate antimicrobial efficacy and safety following topical application of DPK-060*. Accessed June 22, 2020. Available from: https://www.clinicaltrials.gov/ct2/show/study/NCT01522391?term=DPK-060&draw=2&rank=2.

[25] Hon, K. L., Leung, A. K., and Barankin, B. (2013). Barrier repair therapy in atopic dermatitis: an overview. *Am J Clin Dermatol*, 14(5):389-399.

[26] Nathan, S. T., *Identifier NCT00883311. A study of BRT-FC-83C for the treatment of atopic dermatitis*. Accessed June 22, 2020. Available from: https://clinicaltrials.gov/ct2/show/NCT00883311?term=NCT00883311&draw=2&rank=1

[27] Syd, D., *Identifier NCT01826461. An evaluation of PDI-192 0.1% in comparison to PDI-192 0.15% in the treatment of mild to moderate atopic dermatitis*. Accessed June 22, 2020. Available from:

https://www.clinicaltrials.gov/ct2/show/NCT01826461?term=NCT01826461&draw=2&rank=1.

[28] Binu, A., *Identifier NCT03002571. Efficacy and safety of IDP-124 lotion.* Accessed June 22, 2020. Available from: https://www.clinicaltrials.gov/ct2/show/NCT03002571?term=NCT03002571&draw=2&rank=1.

[29] Anya, L., *Identifier NCT03058783. Efficacy and safety of IDP-124 lotion for the treatment of moderate to severe atopic dermatitis in pediatric and adult subjects.* Accessed June 22, 2020. Available from: https://www.clinicaltrials.gov/ct2/show/NCT03058783?term=NCT03058783&draw=2&rank=1.

[30] Claudia, G., *Identifier NCT03795506. TLA in children with moderate to severe atopic eczema (TLA4AE).* Accessed June 22, 2020. Available from: https://www.clinicaltrials.gov/ct2/show/NCT03795506?term=NCT03795506&draw=2&rank=1.

[31] Gandhi, N. A., Bennett, B. L., Graham, N. M., Pirozzi, G., Stahl, N., and Yancopoulos, G. D. (2016). Targeting key proximal drivers of type 2 inflammation in disease. *Nat Rev Drug Discov*, 15(1):35-50.

[32] Gandhi, N. A., Pirozzi, G., and Graham, N. M. (2017). Commonality of the IL-4/IL-13 pathway in atopic diseases. *Expert Rev Clin Immunol*,13(5):425-437.

[33] Hamilton, J. D., Suárez-Fariñas, M., Dhingra, N., Cardinale, I., Li, X., Kostic, A., Ming, J. E., Radin, A. R., Krueger, J. G., Graham, N., Yancopoulos, G. D., Pirozzi, G., and Guttman-Yassky, E. (2014). Dupilumab improves the molecular signature in skin of patients with moderate-to-severe atopic dermatitis. *J Allergy Clin Immunol*, 134(6):1293-1300.

[34] Simpson, E. L., Bieber, T., Guttman-Yassky, E., Beck, L. A., Blauvelt, A., Cork, M. J., Silverberg, J. I., Deleuran, M., Kataoka, Y., Lacour, J. P., Kingo, K., Worm, M., Poulin, Y., Wollenberg, A., Soo, Y., Graham, N. M., Pirozzi, G., Akinlade, B., Staudinger, H., Mastey, V., Eckert, L., Gadkari, A., Stahl, N., Yancopoulos, G. D., Ardeleanu, M., and SOLO 1 and SOLO 2 Investigators (2016). Two

Phase 3 Trials of Dupilumab versus Placebo in Atopic Dermatitis. *N Engl J Med*, 375(24):2335-2348.

[35] Blauvelt, A., de Bruin-Weller, M., Gooderham, M., Cather, J. C., Weisman, J., Pariser, D., Simpson, E. L., Papp, K. A., Hong, H. C., Rubel, D., Foley, P., Prens, E., Griffiths, C., Etoh, T., Pinto, P. H., Pujol, R. M., Szepietowski, J. C., Ettler, K., Kemény, L., Zhu, X., Akinlade, B., Hultsch, T., Mastey, V., Gadkari, A., Eckert, L., Amin, N., Graham, N., Pirozzi, G., Stahl, N., Yancopoulos, G. D., and Shumel, B. (2017). Long-term management of moderate-to-severe atopic dermatitis with dupilumab and concomitant topical corticosteroids (LIBERTY AD CHRONOS): a 1-year, randomised, double-blinded, placebo-controlled, phase 3 trial. *Lancet*, 389 (10086):2287-2303.

[36] Merola, J. F., Sidbury, R., Wollenberg, A., Chen, Z., Zhang, A., Shumel, B., and Rossi, A. B. (2020). Dupilumab prevents flares in adults with moderate-to-severe atopic dermatitis in a 52-week randomized controlled phase 3 trial. *J Am Acad Dermatol*. Accessed June 22, 2020. S0190-9622(20)30822-7. doi: 10.1016/j.jaad.2020.05.003

[37] Silverberg, J. I., Yosipovitch, G., Simpson, E. L., Kim, B. S., Wu, J. J., Eckert, L., Guillemin, I., Chen, Z., Ardeleanu, M., Bansal, A., Kaur, M., Rossi, A. B., Graham, N., Patel, N., and Gadkari, A. (2020). Dupilumab treatment results in early and sustained improvements in itch in adolescents and adults with moderate to severe atopic dermatitis: Analysis of the randomized phase 3 studies SOLO 1 and SOLO 2, AD ADOL, and CHRONOS. *J Am Acad Dermatol*. Accessed June 22, 2020. pii: S0190-9622(20)30305-4.

[38] Tina, B., *Identifier NCT03667014. The impact of dupilumab on quality of life in moderate to severe atopic dermatitis patients.* Accessed June 22, 2020. Available from: https://www.clinicaltrials.gov/ct2/show/NCT03667014?term=NCT03667014&draw=2&rank=1.

[39] Sanofi, *Identifier NCT04033367. SAR231893-LPS15497-"dupilumab effect on sleep in AD patients"*. Accessed June 22, 2020.

Available from: https://www.clinicaltrials.gov/ct2/show/NCT04033367?term=NCT04033367&draw=2&rank=1.

[40] Nutten, S. (2015). Atopic dermatitis: global epidemiology and risk factors. *Ann Nutr Metab*, 66 Suppl 1:8-16.

[41] Simpson, E. L., Paller, A. S., Siegfried, E. C., Boguniewicz, M., Sher, L., Gooderham, M. J., Beck, L. A., Guttman-Yassky, E., Pariser, D., Blauvelt, A., Weisman, J., Lockshin, B., Hultsch, T., Zhang, Q., Kamal, M. A., Davis, J. D., Akinlade, B., Staudinger, H., Hamilton, J. D., Graham, N., Pirozzi, G., Gadkari, A., Eckert, L., Stahl, N., Yancopoulos, G. D., Ruddy, M., and Bansal, A. (2019). Efficacy and safety of dupilumab in adolescents with uncontrolled moderate to severe atopic dermatitis: a phase 3 randomized clinical trial. *JAMA Dermatol*. Accessed June 22, 2020. doi: 10.1001/jamadermatol.2019.3336.

[42] Regeneron Pharma, *Identifier NCT03050151. Study of dupilumab auto-injector device when used by patients with atopic dermatitis*. Accessed June 22, 2020. Available from: https://www.clinicaltrials.gov/ct2/show/NCT03050151?term=NCT03050151&draw=2&rank=1.

[43] de Bruin-Weller, M., Thaçi, D., Smith, C. H., Reich, K., Cork, M. J., Radin, A., Zhang, Q., Akinlade, B., Gadkari, A., Eckert, L., Hultsch, T., Chen, Z., Pirozzi, G., Graham, N., and Shumel, B. (2018). Dupilumab with concomitant topical corticosteroid treatment in adults with atopic dermatitis with an inadequate response or intolerance to ciclosporin A or when this treatment is medically inadvisable: a placebo-controlled, randomized phase III clinical trial (LIBERTY AD CAFÉ). *Br J Dermatol*, 178(5):1083-1101.

[44] Darren, W. and Richard, G., *Identifier NCT00676884. A phase 2a study to investigate the effects of repeated administration of AeroDerm in subjects with atopic eczema*. Accessed June 22, 2020. Available from: https://www.clinicaltrials.gov/ct2/show/NCT00676884?term=NCT00676884&draw=2&rank=1.

[45] Wollenberg, A., Howell, M. D., Guttman-Yassky, E., Silverberg, J. I., Kell, C., Ranade, K., Moate, R., and van der Merwe, R. (2019).

Treatment of atopic dermatitis with tralokinumab, an anti-IL-13 mAb. *J Allergy Clin Immunol*, 143(1):135-141.

[46] LEO Pharma, *Identifier NCT03526861. Tralokinumab monotherapy for adolescent subjects with moderate to severe atopic dermatitis - ECZTRA 6 (ECZema TRAlokinumab Trial no. 6).* Accessed June 22, 2020. Available from: https://www.clinicaltrials.gov/ct2/show/NCT03526861?term=NCT03526861&draw=1&rank=1.

[47] LEO Pharma, *Identifier NCT03587805. Long-term extension trial in subjects with atopic dermatitis who participated in previous tralokinumab trials – ECZTEND.* Accessed June 22, 2020. Available from: https://www.clinicaltrials.gov/ct2/show/NCT03587805?term=NCT03587805&draw=2&rank=1.

[48] Simpson, E. L., Flohr, C., Eichenfield, L. F., Bieber, T., Sofen, H., Taïeb, A., Owen, R., Putnam, W., Castro, M., DeBusk, K., Lin, C. Y., Voulgari, A., Yen, K., and Omachi, T. A. (2018). Efficacy and safety of lebrikizumab (an anti-IL-13 monoclonal antibody) in adults with moderate-to-severe atopic dermatitis inadequately controlled by topical corticosteroids: a randomized, placebo-controlled phase II trial (TREBLE). *J Am Acad Dermatol*, 78(5):863-871.

[49] Guttman-Yassky, E., Blauvelt, A., Eichenfield, L. F., Paller, A. S., Armstrong, A. W., Drew, J., Gopalan, R., and Simpson, E. L. (2020). Efficacy and safety of lebrikizumab, a high-affinity interleukin 13 inhibitor, in adults with moderate to severe atopic dermatitis: a phase 2b randomized clinical trial. *JAMA Dermatol*. Accessed June 22, 2020. doi: 10.1001/jamadermatol.

[50] Wollenberg, A., Howell, M. D., Guttman-Yassky, E., Silverberg, J. I., Birrell, C., Chris Kell, Dawson, M., (2017). A phase 2b dose-ranging efficacy and safety study of tralokinumab in adult patients with moderate to severe atopic dermatitis (AD). *J Am Acad Dermatol*, 6(76): AB20.

[51] Hamid, Q., Boguniewicz, M., and Leung, D. (1994). Differential in situ cytokine gene expression in acute versus chronic atopic dermatitis. *J Clin Invest*, 94(2):870-876.

[52] Guttman-Yassky, E., Nograles, K. E., and Krueger, J. G. (2011). Contrasting pathogenesis of atopic dermatitis and psoriasis - Part II: immune cell subsets and therapeutic concepts. J *Allergy and Clin Immunol*, 127(6):1420-1432.

[53] Kondo, S., Yazawa, H., and Jimbow, K. (2001). Reduction of serum interleukin-5 levels reflect clinical improvement in patients with atopic dermatitis. *J Dermatol*, 28(5):237-243.

[54] Brunner, P. M., Leung, D., and Guttman-Yassky, E. (2018). Immunologic, microbial, and epithelial interactions in atopic dermatitis. *Ann Allergy Asthma Immunol*, 120(1):34-41.

[55] Furue, M., Chiba, T., Tsuji, G., Ulzii, D., Kido-Nakahara, M., Nakahara, T., and Kadono, T. (2017). Atopic dermatitis: immune deviation, barrier dysfunction, IgE autoreactivity and new therapies. *Allergol Int*, 66(3):398-403.

[56] Kang, E. G., Narayana, P. K., Pouliquen, I. J., Lopez, M. C., Ferreira-Cornwell, M. C., and Getsy, J. A. (2020). Efficacy and safety of mepolizumab administered subcutaneously for moderate to severe atopic dermatitis. *Allergy*, 75(4):950-953.

[57] Gail, G., *Identifier NCT03563066. Effect of benralizumab in atopic dermatitis.* Accessed June 22, 2020. Available from: https://www.clinicaltrials.gov/ct2/show/NCT03563066?term=NCT03563066&draw=2&rank=1.

[58] Hardman, C., and Ogg, G. (2016). Interleukin-33, friend and foe in type-2 immune responses. *Curr Opin Immunol*, 42:16-24.

[59] Moussion, C., Ortega, N., and Girard, J. P. (2008). The IL-1-like cytokine IL-33 is constitutively expressed in the nucleus of endothelial cells and epithelial cells in vivo: a novel 'alarmin'? *PLoS One*, 3(10): e3331.

[60] Komai-Koma, M., Brombacher, F., Pushparaj, P. N., Arendse, B., McSharry, C., Alexander, J., Chaudhuri, R., Thomson, N. C., McKenzie, A. N., McInnes, I., Liew, F. Y., and Xu, D. (2012). Interleukin-33 amplifies IgE synthesis and triggers mast cell degranulation via interleukin-4 in naive mice. *Allergy*, 67(9):1118-1126.

[61] Huang, Y., and Paul, W. E. (2016), Inflammatory group 2 innate lymphoid cells. *Int Immunol*, 28(1):23-28.

[62] Moro, K., Yamada, T., Tanabe, M., Takeuchi, T., Ikawa, T., Kawamoto, H., Furusawa, J., Ohtani, M., Fujii, H., and Koyasu, S. (2010). Innate production of T(H)2 cytokines by adipose tissue-associated c-Kit (+) Sca-1(+) lymphoid cells. *Nature*, 463(7280):540-544.

[63] Chen, Y. L., Gutowska-Owsiak, D., Hardman, C. S., Westmoreland, M., MacKenzie, T., Cifuentes, L., Waithe, D., Lloyd-Lavery, A., Marquette, A., Londei, M., and Ogg, G. (2019). Proof-of-concept clinical trial of etokimab shows a key role for IL-33 in atopic dermatitis pathogenesis. *Sci Transl Med*,11(515). Accessed June 22, 2020. pii: eaax2945.

[64] Nnane, I., Frederick, B., Yao, Z., Raible, D., Shu, C., Badorrek, P., van den Boer, M., Branigan, P., Duffy, K., Baribaud, F., Fink, D., Yang, T. Y., and Xu, Z. (2020). The first-in-human study of CNTO 7160, an anti-interleukin-33 receptor monoclonal antibody, in healthy subjects and patients with asthma or atopic dermatitis. *Br J Clin Pharmacol*. Accessed June 22, 2020. doi:10.1111/bcp.14361.

[65] Quentmeier, H., Drexler, H. G., Fleckenstein, D., Zaborski, M., Armstrong, A., Sims, J. E., and Lyman, S. D. (2001). Cloning of human thymic stromal lymphopoietin (TSLP) and signaling mechanisms leading to proliferation. *Leukemia*, 15(8):1286-1292.

[66] Verstraete, K., Peelman, F., Braun, H., Lopez, J., Van Rompaey, D., Dansercoer, A., Vandenberghe, I., Pauwels, K., Tavernier, J., Lambrecht, B. N., Hammad, H., De Winter, H., Beyaert, R., Lippens, G., and Savvides, S. N. (2017). Structure and antagonism of the receptor complex mediated by human TSLP in allergy and asthma. *Nat Commun*, 8:14937.

[67] Wang, Q., Du, J., Zhu, J., Yang, X., and Zhou, B. (2015). Thymic stromal lymphopoietin signaling in CD4(+) T cells is required for TH2 memory. *J Allergy Clin Immunol*,135(3):781-791.

[68] Soumelis, V., Reche, P. A., Kanzler, H., Yuan, W., Edward, G., Homey, B., Gilliet, M., Ho, S., Antonenko, S., Lauerma, A., Smith,

K., Gorman, D., Zurawski, S., Abrams, J., Menon, S., McClanahan, T., de Waal-Malefyt Rd, R., Bazan, F., Kastelein, R. A., and Liu, Y. J. (2002). Human epithelial cells trigger dendritic cell mediated allergic inflammation by producing TSLP. *Nat Immunol*, 3(7):673-680.

[69] Bell, B. D., Kitajima, M., Larson, R. P., Stoklasek, T. A., Dang, K., Sakamoto, K., Wagner, K. U., Kaplan, D. H., Reizis, B., Hennighausen, L., and Ziegler, S. F. (2013). The transcription factor STAT5 is critical in dendritic cells for the development of TH2 but not TH1 responses. *Nat Immunol*,14(4):364-371.

[70] Parnes, J. R., Sullivan, J. T., Chen, L., and Dias, C. (2019). Pharmacokinetics, safety, and tolerability of tezepelumab (AMG 157) in healthy and atopic dermatitis adult subjects. *Clin Pharmacol Ther*, 106(2):441-449.

[71] Simpson, E. L., Parnes, J. R., She, D., Crouch, S., Rees, W., Mo, M., and van der Merwe, R. (2019). Tezepelumab, an anti-thymic stromal lymphopoietin monoclonal antibody, in the treatment of moderate to severe atopic dermatitis: A randomized phase 2a clinical trial. *J Am Acad Dermatol*,80(4):1013-1021.

[72] Numazaki, M., Hanaoka, K., Imamura, E., Maeda, M., Arai, K., Saito, T., Takamura, F., Suzuki H., Kubo, S., and Furukawa, S., (2018). ASP7266, a novel antibody against human TSLPR, in the treatment of allergic disease. *J Allergy Clin Immunol Pract*, 141(2), suppl, AB13.

[73] Chung, K. F. (2015). Targeting the interleukin pathway in the treatment of asthma. *Lancet*, 386(9998):1086-1096.

[74] Wu, A. C. (2019). Omalizumab for atopic dermatitis: over-treatment or lifesaver? *JAMA Pediatr*. Accessed June 22, 2020. doi: 10.1001/jamapediatrics.2019.4509.

[75] Chan, S., Cornelius, V., Cro, S., Harper, J. I., and Lack, G. (2019). *JAMA Pediatr*. Accessed June 22, 2020. doi: 10.1001/jamapediatrics. 2019.4476.

[76] Slomski, A. (2020). Anti-IgE medication lessens pediatric atopic dermatitis severity. *JAMA*, 323(8):701.

[77] Zink, A., Gensbaur, A., Zirbs, M., Seifert, F., Suarez, I. L., Mourantchanian, V., Weidinger, S., Mempel, M., Ring, J., and Ollert, M. (2016). Targeting IgE in severe atopic dermatitis with a combination of immunoadsorption and omalizumab. *Acta Derm Venereol*, 96(1):72-76.

[78] Sheldon, E., Schwickart, M., Li, J., Kim, K., Crouch, S., Parveen, S., Kell, C., and Birrell, C. (2016). Pharmacokinetics, pharmacodynamics, and safety of MEDI4212, an anti-IgE monoclonal antibody, in subjects with atopy: a phase I study. *Adv Ther*, 33(2), 225–251.

[79] Novartis Pharma, *Identifier NCT01552629. A study evaluating the safety and efficacy of QGE031 in atopic dermatitis patients. Accessed June 22, 2020.* Available from: https://www.clinicaltrials.gov/ct2/show/NCT01552629?term=NCT01552629&draw=2&rank=1.

[80] Novartis Pharma, *Identifier NCT01596712. Safety, tolerability, pharmacokinetics, pharmacodynamics and immunogenicity of QGE031 in Japanese atopic male subjects.* Accessed June 22, 2020. Available from: https://www.clinicaltrials.gov/ct2/show/NCT01596712?term=NCT01596712&draw=2&rank=1.

[81] Noda, S., Suárez-Fariñas, M., Ungar, B., Kim, S. J., de Guzman Strong, C., Xu, H., Peng, X., Estrada, Y. D., Nakajima, S., Honda, T., Shin, J. U., Lee, H., Krueger, J. G., Lee, K. H., Kabashima, K., and Guttman-Yassky, E. (2015). The Asian atopic dermatitis phenotype combines features of atopic dermatitis and psoriasis with increased TH17 polarization. *J Allergy Clin Immunol*, 136(5):1254-1264.

[82] Eyerich, K., Pennino, D., Scarponi, C., Foerster, S., Nasorri, F., Behrendt, H., Ring, J., Traidl-Hoffmann, C., Albanesi, C., and Cavani, A. (2009). IL-17 in atopic eczema: linking allergen-specific adaptive and microbial-triggered innate immune response. *J Allergy Clin Immunol*, 123(1):59-66.

[83] Li, J., Leyva-Castillo, J. M., Hener, P., Eisenmann, A., Zaafouri, S., Jonca, N., Serre, G., Birling, M. C., and Li, M. (2016). Counterregulation between thymic stromal lymphopoietin- and IL-

23-driven immune axes shapes skin inflammation in mice with epidermal barrier defects. *J Allergy Clin Immunol*, 138(1):150-161.

[84] Nograles, K. E., Zaba, L. C., Shemer, A., Fuentes-Duculan, J., Cardinale, I., Kikuchi, T., Ramon, M., Bergman, R., Krueger, J. G., and Guttman-Yassky, E. (2009). IL-22-producing "T22" T cells account for upregulated IL-22 in atopic dermatitis despite reduced IL-17-producing TH17 T cells. *J Allergy Clin Immunol*, 123(6):1244-1252.

[85] Czarnowicki, T., Gonzalez, J., Shemer, A., Malajian, D., Xu, H., Zheng, X., Khattri, S., Gilleaudeau, P., Sullivan-Whalen, M., Suárez-Fariñas, M., Krueger, J. G., and Guttman-Yassky, E. (2015). Severe atopic dermatitis is characterized by selective expansion of circulating TH2/TC2 and TH22/TC22, but not TH17/TC17, cells within the skin-homing T-cell population. *J Allergy Clin Immunol*, 136(1):104–115.

[86] Gittler, J. K., Shemer, A., Suárez-Fariñas, M., Fuentes-Duculan, J., Gulewicz, K. J., Wang, C. Q., Mitsui, H., Cardinale, I., de Guzman Strong, C., Krueger, J. G., and Guttman-Yassky, E. (2012). Progressive activation of T(H)2/T(H)22 cytokines and selective epidermal proteins characterizes acute and chronic atopic dermatitis. *J Allergy Clin Immunol*, 130(6):1344–1354.

[87] Noda, S., Hashim, P. W., Khattri, S., Shroff, A., and Guttman-Yassky, E. (2016). Successful use of secukinumab in an Asian patient with severe refractory atopic dermatitis. *J Invest Dermatol*, 136(5), S40.

[88] Ungar, B., Pavel, A. B., Li, R., Kimmel, G., Nia, J., Hashim, P., Kim, H. J., Chima, M., Vekaria, A. S., Estrada, Y., Xu, H., Peng, X., Singer, G. K., Baum, D., Mansouri, Y., Taliercio, M., and Guttman-Yassky, E. (2020). Phase 2 randomized, double-blind study of IL-17-targeting with secukinumab in atopic dermatitis. *J Allergy Clin Immunol*, S0091-6749(20)30684-9. doi: 10.1016/j.jaci.2020.04.055

[89] Stefan, B., *Identifier NCT03568136. Investigation of efficacy of secukinumab in patients with moderate to serve atopic dermatitis (Secu_in_AD).* Accessed June 22, 2020. Available from:

https://www.clinicaltrials.gov/ct2/show/NCT03568136?term=NCT03568136&draw=2&rank=1.

[90] Lauffer, F., Jargosch, M., Baghin, V., Krause, L., Kempf, W., Absmaier-Kijak, M., Morelli, M., Madonna, S., Marsais, F., Lepescheux, L., Albanesi, C., Müller, N. S., Theis, F. J., Schmidt-Weber, C., Eyerich, S., Biedermann, T., Vandeghinste, N., Steidl, S., and Eyerich, K. (2020). IL-17C amplifies epithelial inflammation in human psoriasis and atopic eczema. *J Eur Acad Dermatol Venereol*; 34(4):800-809.

[91] Vandeghinste, N., Klattig, J., Jagerschmidt, C., Lavazais, S., Marsais, F., Haas, J. D., Auberval, M., Lauffer, F., Moran, T., Ongenaert, M., Van Balen, M., Dupont, S., Lepescheux, L., Garcia, T., Härtle, S., Eyerich, K., Fallon, P. G., Brys, R., and Steidl, S. (2018). Neutralization of IL-17C reduces skin inflammation in mouse models of psoriasis and atopic dermatitis. *J Invest Dermatol*, 138(7):1555-1563.

[92] Helen, T., *Identifier NCT03568071. A study to assess efficacy, safety, tolerability and pharmacokinetics (PK)/pharmacodynamics (PD) of MOR106 in subjects with moderate to severe atopic dermatitis (IGUANA).* Accessed June 22, 2020. Available from: https://www.clinicaltrials.gov/ct2/show/NCT03568071?term=NCT03568071&draw=2&rank=1.

[93] Helen, T., *Identifier NCT03864627. A study to test safety and tolerability of a study drug called MOR106 administered concomitantly with topical corticosteroids, in adult patients with moderate to severe atopic dermatitis (GECKO).* Accessed June 22, 2020. Available from: https://www.clinicaltrials.gov/ct2/show/NCT03864627?term=NCT03864627&draw=2&rank=1.

[94] Kimball, A. B., Papp, K. A., Wasfi, Y., Chan, D., Bissonnette, R., Sofen, H., Yeilding, N., Li, S., Szapary, P., Gordon, K. B., and PHOENIX 1 Investigators (2013). Long-term efficacy of ustekinumab in patients with moderate-to-severe psoriasis treated for up to 5 years in the PHOENIX 1 study. *J Eur Acad Dermatol Venereol*, 27(12):1535-1545.

[95] Saeki, H., Kabashima, K., Tokura, Y., Murata, Y., Shiraishi, A., Tamamura, R., Randazzo, B., and Imanaka, K. (2017). Efficacy and safety of ustekinumab in Japanese patients with severe atopic dermatitis: a randomized, double-blind, placebo-controlled, phase II study. *Br J Dermatol*, 177(2):419-427.

[96] Guttman-Yassky, E., Brunner, P. M., Neumann, A. U., Khattri, S., Pavel, A. B., Malik, K., Singer, G. K., Baum, D., Gilleaudeau, P., Sullivan-Whalen, M., Rose, S., Jim On, S., Li, X., Fuentes-Duculan, J., Estrada, Y., Garcet, S., Traidl-Hoffmann, C., Krueger, J. G., and Lebwohl, M. G. (2018). Efficacy and safety of fezakinumab (an IL-22 monoclonal antibody) in adults with moderate-to-severe atopic dermatitis inadequately controlled by conventional treatments: a randomized, double-blind, phase 2a trial. *J Am Acad Dermatol*, 78(5):872-881.

[97] Brunner, P. M., Pavel, A. B., Khattri, S., Leonard, A., Malik, K., Rose, S., Jim On, S., Vekaria, A. S., Traidl-Hoffmann, C., Singer, G. K., Baum, D., Gilleaudeau, P., Sullivan-Whalen, M., Fuentes-Duculan, J., Li, X., Zheng, X., Estrada, Y., Garcet, S., Wen, H. C., Gonzalez, J., Coats, I., Cueto, I., Neumann, A. U., Lebwohl, M. G., Krueger, J. G., and Guttman-Yassky, E. (2019). Baseline IL-22 expression in patients with atopic dermatitis stratifies tissue responses to fezakinumab. *J Allergy Clin Immunol*, 143(1):142-154.

[98] Jacobi, A., Antoni, C., Manger, B., Schuler, G., and Hertl, M. (2005). Infliximab in the treatment of moderate to severe atopic dermatitis. *J Am Acad Dermatol*, 52(3 Pt 1):522-526.

[99] Buka, R. L., Resh, B., Roberts, B., Cunningham, B. B., and Friedlander, S. (2005). Etanercept is minimally effective in 2 children with atopic dermatitis. *J Am Acad Dermatol*, 53(2):358-359.

[100] Guttman-Yassky, E., Pavel, A. B., Zhou, L., et al. (2019). GBR 830, an anti-OX40, improves skin gene signatures and clinical scores in patients with atopic dermatitis. *J Allergy Clin Immunol*, 144(2):482-493.

[101] Andrea, A., *Identifier NCT03568162. Phase 2b study to evaluate the efficacy and safety of ISB 830 in adults with moderate to severe*

atopic dermatitis. Accessed June 22, 2020. Available from: https://www.clinicaltrials.gov/ct2/show/NCT03568162?term=NCT03568162&draw=2&rank=1.

[102] Stephan, W., *Identifier NCT03754309. A study of KY1005 in patients with moderate to severe atopic dermatitis.* Accessed June 22, 2020. Available from: https://www.clinicaltrials.gov/ct2/show/NCT03754309?term=NCT03754309&draw=2&rank=1.

[103] Ehsanollah, E., *Identifier NCT03703102. Study of an anti-OX40 monoclonal antibody (KHK4083) in subjects with moderate to severe atopic dermatitis.* Accessed June 22, 2020. Available from: https://www.clinicaltrials.gov/ct2/show/NCT03703102?term=NCT03703102&draw=2&rank=1.

[104] Kim, H. O., Kim, J. H., Chung, B. Y., Choi, M. G., and Park, C. W. (2014). *Increased expression of the aryl hydrocarbon receptor in patients with chronic inflammatory skin diseases. Exp Dermatol,* 23(4):278-281.

[105] Smith, S. H., Jayawickreme, C., Rickard, D. J., Nicodeme, E., Bui, T., Simmons, C., Coquery, C. M., Neil, J., Pryor, W. M., Mayhew, D., Rajpal, D. K., Creech, K., Furst, S., Lee, J., Wu, D., Rastinejad, F., Willson, T. M., Viviani, F., Morris, D. C., Moore, J. T., and Cote-Sierra, J. (2017). Tapinarof is a natural AhR agonist that resolves skin inflammation in mice and humans. *J Invest Dermatol,* 137(10):2110-2119.

[106] van den Bogaard, E. H., Bergboer, J. G., Vonk-Bergers, M., van Vlijmen-Willems, I. M., Hato, S. V., van der Valk, P. G., Schröder, J. M., Joosten, I., Zeeuwen, P. L., and Schalkwijk, J. (2013). Coal tar induces AHR-dependent skin barrier repair in atopic dermatitis. *J Clin Invest,* 123(2):917-927.

[107] Bissonnette, R., Chen, G., Bolduc, C., Maari, C., Lyle, M., Tang, L., Webster, J., and Zhou, Y. (2010). Efficacy and safety of topical WBI-1001 in the treatment of atopic dermatitis: results from a phase 2A, randomized, placebo-controlled clinical trial. *Arch Dermatol,* 146(4):446-449.

[108] Bissonnette, R., Poulin, Y., Zhou, Y., Tan, J., Hong, H. C., Webster, J., Ip, W., Tang, L., and Lyle, M. (2012). Efficacy and safety of topical WBI-1001 in patients with mild to severe atopic dermatitis: results from a 12-week, multicentre, randomized, placebo-controlled double-blind trial. *Br J Dermatol*, 166(4):853-860.

[109] Peppers, J., Paller, A. S., Maeda-Chubachi, T., Wu, S., Robbins, K., Gallagher, K., and Kraus, J. E. (2019). A phase 2, randomized dose-finding study of tapinarof (GSK2894512 cream) for the treatment of atopic dermatitis. *J Am Acad Dermatol*, 80(1):89-98.

[110] Paller, A. S., Gold, L. S., Soung, J., Tallman, A. M., Rubenstein, D. S., and Gooderham, M. (2020). Efficacy and patient-reported outcomes from a phase IIb, randomized clinical trial of tapinarof cream for the treatment of adolescents and adults with atopic dermatitis. *J Am Acad Dermatol*, S0190-9622(20)31011-2. Accessed June 22, 2020. doi. 10.1016/j.jaad.2020.05.135.

[111] Serezani, C. H., Ballinger, M. N., Aronoff, D. M., and Peters-Golden, M. (2008). Cyclic AMP: master regulator of innate immune cell function. *Am J Respir Cell Mol Biol*, 39(2), 127–132.

[112] Butler, J. M., Chan, S. C., Stevens, S., and Hanifin, J. M. (1983). Increased leukocyte histamine release with elevated cyclic AMP-phosphodiesterase activity in atopic dermatitis. *J Allergy Clin Immunol*, 71(5):490-497.

[113] Hanifin, J. M., Chan, S. C., Cheng, J. B., Tofte, S. J., Henderson, W. R., Jr, Kirby, D. S., and Weiner, E. S. (1996). Type 4 phosphodiesterase inhibitors have clinical and in vitro anti-inflammatory effects in atopic dermatitis. *J Invest Dermatol*, 107(1): 51-56.

[114] Paller, A. S., Tom, W. L., Lebwohl, M. G., Blumenthal, R. L., Boguniewicz, M., Call, R. S., Eichenfield, L. F., Forsha, D. W., Rees, W. C., Simpson, E. L., Spellman, M. C., Stein Gold, L. F., Zaenglein, A. L., Hughes, M. H., Zane, L. T., and Hebert, A. A. (2016). Efficacy and safety of crisaborole ointment, a novel, nonsteroidal phosphodiesterase 4 (PDE4) inhibitor for the topical treatment of

atopic dermatitis (AD) in children and adults. *J Am Acad Dermatol*, 75(3):494-503.

[115] Nemoto, O., Hayashi, N., Kitahara, Y., Furue, M., Hojo, S., Nomoto, M., Shima, S., and Japanese E6005 Study Investigators (2016). Effect of topical phosphodiesterase 4 inhibitor E6005 on Japanese children with atopic dermatitis: results from a randomized, vehicle-controlled exploratory trial. *J Dermatol*, 43(8):881-887.

[116] Ohba, F., Nomoto, M., Hojo, S., and Akama, H. (2016). Safety, tolerability and pharmacokinetics of a novel phosphodiesterase inhibitor, E6005 ointment, in healthy volunteers and in patients with atopic dermatitis. *J Dermatolog Treat*, 27(3):241-246.

[117] Kitahara, Y., Hojo, S., Nomoto, M., Onozuka, D., Furue, M., and Hagihara, A. (2019). Pharmacokinetic disposition of topical phosphodiesterase-4 inhibitor E6005 in patients with atopic dermatitis. *J Dermatolog Treat*, 30(5):466-470.

[118] Hanifin, J. M., Ellis, C. N., Frieden, I. J., Fölster-Holst, R., Stein Gold, L. F., Secci, A., Smith, A. J., Zhao, C., Kornyeyeva, E., and Eichenfield, L. F. (2016). OPA-15406, a novel, topical, nonsteroidal, selective phosphodiesterase-4 (PDE4) inhibitor, in the treatment of adult and adolescent patients with mild to moderate atopic dermatitis (AD): a phase-II randomized, double-blind, placebo-controlled study. *J Am Acad Dermatol*, 75(2):297-305.

[119] Saeki, H., Baba, N., Oshiden, K., Abe, Y., and Tsubouchi, H. (2020). Phase 2, randomized, double-blind, placebo-controlled, 4-week study to evaluate the safety and efficacy of OPA- 15406 (difamilast), a new topical selective phosphodiesterase type-4 inhibitor, in Japanese pediatric patients aged 2-14 years with atopic dermatitis. *J Dermatol*, 47(1):17-24.

[120] Felding, J., Sørensen, M. D., Poulsen, T. D., Larsen, J., Andersson, C., Refer, P., Engell, K., Ladefoged, L. G., Thormann, T., Vinggaard, A. M., Hegardt, P., Søhoel, A., and Nielsen, S. F. (2014). Discovery and early clinical development of 2-{6-[2-(3,5-dichloro-4-pyridyl) acetyl]-2,3-dimethoxyphenoxy}-N-propylacetamide (LEO 29102), a

soft-drug inhibitor of phosphodiesterase 4 for topical treatment of atopic dermatitis. *J Med Chem*, 57(14):5893-5903.

[121] Beth, Z., *Identifier NCT01993420. A safety and efficacy of DRM02 in subjects with atopic dermatitis*. Accessed June 22, 2020. Available from: https://www.clinicaltrials.gov/ct2/show/NCT01993420?term=NCT01993420&draw=2&rank=1.

[122] Schwartz, D. M., Kanno, Y., Villarino, A., Ward, M., Gadina, M., and O'Shea, J. J. (2017). JAK inhibition as a therapeutic strategy for immune and inflammatory diseases. *Nat Rev Drug Discov*, 17(1):78.

[123] Howell, M. D., Fitzsimons, C., and Smith, P. (2018). JAK/STAT inhibitors and other small molecule cytokine antagonists for the treatment of allergic disease. *Ann Allergy Asthma Immunol*, 120(4):367e375.

[124] Bissonnette, R., Papp, K. A., Poulin, Y., Gooderham, M., Raman, M., Mallbris, L., Wang, C., Purohit, V., Mamolo, C., Papacharalambous, J., and Ports, W. C. (2016). Topical tofacitinib for atopic dermatitis: a phase IIa randomized trial. *Br J Dermatol*, 175(5):902–911.

[125] Levy, L. L., Urban, J., and King, B. A. (2015). Treatment of recalcitrant atopic dermatitis with the oral Janus kinase inhibitor tofacitinib citrate. *J Am Acad Dermatol*, 73(3):395–399.

[126] Nakagawa, H., Nemoto, O., Yamada, H., Nagata, T., and Ninomiya, N. (2018). Phase 1 studies to assess the safety, tolerability and pharmacokinetics of JTE-052 (a novel Janus kinase inhibitor) ointment in Japanese healthy volunteers and patients with atopic dermatitis. *J Dermatol*, 45(6):701-709.

[127] Nakagawa, H., Nemoto, O., Igarashi, A., and Nagata, T. (2018). Efficacy and safety of topical JTE-052, a Janus kinase inhibitor, in Japanese adult patients with moderate-to-severe atopic dermatitis: a phase II, multicentre, randomized, vehicle-controlled clinical study. *Br J Dermatol*, 178(2):424-432.

[128] Guttman-Yassky, E., Silverberg, J. I., Nemoto, O., Forman, S. B., Wilke, A., Prescilla, R., de la Peña, A., Nunes, F. P., Janes, J., Gamalo, M., Donley, D., Paik, J., DeLozier, A. M., Nickoloff, B. J.,

and Simpson, E. L. (2019). Baricitinib in adult patients with moderate-to-severe atopic dermatitis: A phase 2 parallel, double-blinded, randomized placebo-controlled multiple-dose study. *J Am Acad Dermatol*, 80(4):913-921.

[129] Simpson, E. L., Lacour, J. P., Spelman, L., Galimberti, R., Eichenfield, L. F., Bissonnette, R., King, B. A., Thyssen, J. P., Silverberg, J. I., Bieber, T., Kabashima, K., Tsunemi, Y., Costanzo, A., Guttman-Yassky, E., Beck, L. A., Janes, J. M., DeLozier, A. M., Gamalo, M., Brinker, D. R., Cardillo, T., Nunes, F. P., Paller, A. S., Wollenberg, A., Reich, K. (2020). Baricitinib in patients with moderate-to-severe atopic dermatitis and inadequate response to topical corticosteroids: results from two randomized monotherapy phase III trials. *Br J Dermatol*. Accessed June 22, 2020. doi: 10.1111/bjd.18898.

[130] Kunwar, S., Collins, C. E., and Constantinescu, F. (2018). Baricitinib, a Janus kinase inhibitor, in the treatment of rheumatoid arthritis: a systematic literature review and meta-analysis of randomized controlled trials. *Clin Rheumatol*, 37(10): 2611-2620.

[131] Kim, B. S., Sun, K., Papp, K., Venturanza, M., Nasir, A., and Kuligowski, M. E. (2020). Effects of ruxolitinib cream on pruritus and quality of life in atopic dermatitis: results from a phase 2, randomized, dose-ranging, vehicle- and active-controlled study. *J Am Acad Dermatol*. pii: S0190-9622(20)30213-9. Accessed June 22, 2020. doi: 10.1016/j.jaad.2020.02.009.

[132] Kim, B. S., Howell, M. D., Sun, K., Papp, K., Nasir, A., Kuligowski, M. E., & INCB 18424-206 Study Investigators (2020). Treatment of atopic dermatitis with ruxolitinib cream (JAK1/JAK2 inhibitor) or triamcinolone cream. *J Allergy Clin Immunol*, 145(2):572-582.

[133] Michael, E. K., *Identifier NCT03745651. TRuE AD2 - an efficacy and safety study of ruxolitinib cream in adolescents and adults with atopic dermatitis.* Accessed June 22, 2020. Available from: https://www.clinicaltrials.gov/ct2/show/NCT03745651?term=NCT03745651&draw=2&rank=1.

[134] Michael, E. K., *Identifier NCT03745638. TRuE AD1 - an efficacy and safety study of ruxolitinib cream in adolescents and adults with atopic dermatitis.* Accessed June 22, 2020. Available from: https://www.clinicaltrials.gov/ct2/show/NCT03745638?term=NCT03745638&draw=2&rank=1.

[135] Michael, K., *Identifier NCT03257644. A pharmacokinetic study of ruxolitinib phosphate cream in pediatric subjects with atopic dermatitis*. Accessed June 22, 2020. Available from: https://www.clinicaltrials.gov/ct2/show/NCT03257644?term=NCT03257644&draw=2&rank=1.

[136] Gooderham, M. J., Forman, S. B., Bissonnette, R., Beebe, J. S., Zhang, W., Banfield, C., Zhu, L., Papacharalambous, J., Vincent, M. S., and Peeva, E. (2019). Efficacy and safety of oral Janus Kinase 1 inhibitor abrocitinib for patients with atopic dermatitis: a phase 2 randomized clinical trial. *JAMA Dermatol*. Accessed June 22, 2020. doi: 10.1001/jamadermatol.2019.2855.

[137] Silverberg, J. I., Simpson, E. L., Thyssen, J. P., Gooderham, M., Chan, G., Feeney, C., Biswas, P., Valdez, H., DiBonaventura, M., Nduaka, C., & Rojo, R. (2020). Efficacy and safety of abrocitinib in patients with moderate-to-severe atopic dermatitis: a randomized clinical trial. *JAMA Dermatol*. Accessed June 22, 2020. doi: 10.1001/jamadermatol.2020.1406.

[138] Guttman-Yassky, E., Thaçi, D., Pangan, A. L., Hong, H. C., Papp, K. A., Reich, K., Beck, L. A., Mohamed, M. F., Othman, A. A., Anderson, J. K., Gu, Y., Teixeira, H. D., and Silverberg, J. I. (2020). Upadacitinib in adults with moderate to severe atopic dermatitis: 16-week results from a randomized, placebo-controlled trial. *J Allergy Clin Immunol*, 145(3):877-884.

[139] Jianzhong, Z., *Identifier NCT04162899. A phase II study in adult patients with moderate to severe atopic dermatitis*. Accessed June 22, 2020. Available from: https://www.clinicaltrials.gov/ct2/show/NCT04162899?term=NCT04162899&draw=2&rank=1.

[140] Glatzer, F., Gschwandtner, M., Ehling, S., Rossbach, K., Janik, K., Klos, A., Bäumer, W., Kietzmann, M., Werfel, T., and Gutzmer, R.

(2013). Histamine induces proliferation in keratinocytes from patients with atopic dermatitis through the histamine 4 receptor. *J Allergy Clin Immunol*. 132(6):1358-1367.

[141] Miyano, K., Matsushita, S., Tsuchida, T., and Nakamura, K. (2016). Inhibitory effect of a histamine 4 receptor antagonist on CCL17 and CCL22 production by monocytederived Langerhans cells in patients with atopic dermatitis. *J Dermatol*, 43(9):1024-1029.

[142] De Benedetto, A., Yoshida, T., Fridy, S., Park, J. E., Kuo, I. H., and Beck, L. A. (2015). Histamine and skin barrier: are histamine antagonists useful for the prevention or treatment of atopic dermatitis? *J Clin Med*, 4(4):741-755.

[143] Werfel, T., Layton, G., Yeadon, M., Whitlock, L., Osterloh, I., Jimenez, P., Liu, W., Lynch, V., Asher, A., Tsianakas, A., and Purkins, L. (2019). Efficacy and safety of the histamine H4 receptor antagonist ZPL-3893787 in patients with atopic dermatitis. *J Allergy Clin Immunol*, 143(5):1830-1837.

[144] Novartis Pharm, *Identifier NCT03948334. A study to assess the safety and efficacy of ZPL389 with TCS/TCI in atopic dermatitis patients (ZESTExt).* Accessed June 22, 2020. Available from: https://www.clinicaltrials.gov/ct2/show/NCT03948334?term=NCT03948334&draw=2&rank=1.

[145] Perez, E., Voronkov, M., Fernandez, J. R., Feng, X., Rounzard, K., Stork, M., Gordon, J. S., Stork, J. B., and Shroot, B. (2011). Preclinical anti-inflammatory activity and safety assessment of SIG990, a novel topical small molecule for the treatment of rosacea. *The 70th Annual Meeting of the Society of Investigative Dermatology*. Poster presentation.

[146] Palmqvist, N., Siller, M., Klint, C., and Sjodin, A. (2016). A human and animal model-based approach to investigating the anti-inflammatory profile and potential of the 5-HT2B receptor antagonist AM1030. *J Inflamm (Lond)*, 13:20.

[147] Christopher, N., Identifier NCT02949960. DMT210 topical gel in the treatment of atopic dermatitis. Accessed June 22, 2020. Available

from: https://www.clinicaltrials.gov/ct2/show/NCT02949960?term=NCT02949960&draw=2&rank=1.

[148] Jim, B., *Identifier NCT02379910. A study to assess the safety, tolerability, PK and PD of AM1030-CREAM in patients with atopic dermatitis.* Accessed June 22, 2020. Available from: https://www.clinicaltrials.gov/ct2/show/NCT02379910?term=NCT02379910&draw=2&rank=1.

[149] Qurient Co., *Identifier NCT02426359. Safety and efficacy study of Q301 in moderate to severe atopic dermatitis patients.* Accessed June 22, 2020. Available from: https://www.clinicaltrials.gov/ct2/show/NCT02426359?term=NCT02426359&draw=2&rank=1.

[150] Qurient Co., *Identifier NCT03571620. Safety and efficacy study of Q301 in mild to moderate adolescents and adults atopic dermatitis patients.* Accessed June 22, 2020. Available from: https://www.clinicaltrials.gov/ct2/show/NCT03571620?term=NCT03571620&draw=2&rank=1.

[151] LEO Pharma., *Identifier NCT02496546. An explorative trial evaluating the effect of LEO 32731 cream in adults with mild to moderate atopic dermatitis (AD).* Accessed June 22, 2020. Available from: https://www.clinicaltrials.gov/ct2/show/NCT02496546?term=NCT02496546&draw=2&rank=1.

[152] Lydia, G., *Identifier NCT02219633. Effect of LEO 39652 cream in adults with mild to moderate atopic dermatitis (AD).* Accessed June 22, 2020. Available from: https://www.clinicaltrials.gov/ct2/show/NCT02219633?term=NCT02219633&draw=2&rank=1.

[153] Joseph, C., *Identifier NCT01850849. Safety, tolerability and pharmacokinetics in AD subjects and healthy subjects of cutaneous application of LEO 39652 cream.* Accessed June 22, 2020. Available from: https://www.clinicaltrials.gov/ct2/show/NCT01850849?term=NCT01850849&draw=2&rank=1.

[154] Yang, T. B., Kim, B. S. (2019). Pruritus in allergy and immunology. *J Allergy Clin Immunol*, 144(2):353-360.

[155] Nakajima, S., Nomura, T., Common, J., and Kabashima, K. (2019). Insights into atopic dermatitis gained from genetically defined mouse models. *J Allergy Clin Immunol*, 143(1):13-25.

[156] Mack, M. R., and Kim, B. S. (2018). The itch-scratch cycle: a neuroimmune perspective. *Trends Immunol*, 39(12):980-991.

[157] Silverberg, J. I., Pinter, A., Pulka, G., Poulin, Y., Bouaziz, J. D., Wollenberg, A., Murrell, D. F., Alexis, A., Lindsey, L., Ahmad, F., Piketty, C., and Clucas, A. (2020). Phase 2B randomized study of nemolizumab in adults with moderate-to-severe atopic dermatitis and severe pruritus. *Allergy Clin Immunol*, 145(1):173-182.

[158] Kabashima, K., Furue, M., Hanifin, J. M., Pulka, G., Wollenberg, A., Galus, R., Etoh, T., Mihara, R., Nakano, M., & Ruzicka, T. (2018). Nemolizumab in patients with moderate-to-severe atopic dermatitis: randomized, phase II, long-term extension study. *J Allergy Clin Immunol*, 142(4):1121-1130.

[159] Galderma R&D, *Identifier NCT03921411. A pharmacokinetics and safety study of nemolizumab in adolescent subjects with atopic dermatitis (AD).* Accessed June 22, 2020. Available from: https://www.clinicaltrials.gov/ct2/show/NCT03921411?term=NCT03921411&draw=2&rank=1.

[160] Galderma R&D, *Identifier NCT03989206. Long-term safety and efficacy of nemolizumab with moderate-to-severe atopic dermatitis.* Accessed June 22, 2020.Available from: https://www.clinicaltrials.gov/ct2/show/NCT03989206?term=NCT03989206&draw=2&rank=1.

[161] Galderma R&D, *Identifier NCT03985943. Efficacy and safety of nemolizumab in subjects with moderate-to-severe atopic dermatitis.* Accessed June 22, 2020. Available from: https://www.clinicaltrials.gov/ct2/show/NCT03985943?term=NCT03985943&draw=2&rank=1.

[162] Galderma R&D, *Identifier NCT03989349. Efficacy & safety of nemolizumab in subjects with moderate-to-severe atopic dermatitis.* Accessed June 22, 2020. Available from: https://www.clinicaltrials.

gov/ct2/show/NCT03989349?term=NCT03989349&draw=2&rank =1.

[163] Kobayashi, T., Glatz, M., Horiuchi, K., Kawasaki, H., Akiyama, H., Kaplan, D. H., Kong, H. H., Amagai, M., and Nagao, K. (2015). Dysbiosis and *Staphylococcus aureus* colonization drives inflammation in atopic dermatitis. *Immunity*, 42(4):756-766.

[164] Gueniche, A., Knaudt, B., Schuck, E., Volz, T., Bastien, P., Martin, R., Röcken, M., Breton, L., and Biedermann, T. (2008). Effects of nonpathogenic gram-negative bacterium *Vitreoscilla filiformis* lysate on atopic dermatitis: a prospective, randomized, double-blind, placebo-controlled clinical study. *Br J Dermatol*, 159(6):1357-1363.

[165] Nakatsuji, T., Chen, T. H., Narala, S., Chun, K. A., Two, A. M., Yun, T., Shafiq, F., Kotol, P. F., Bouslimani, A., Melnik, A. V., Latif, H., Kim, J. N., Lockhart, A., Artis, K., David, G., Taylor, P., Streib, J., Dorrestein, P. C., Grier, A., Gill, S. R., Zengler K, Hata TR, Leung DY, Gallo, R. L. (2017). Antimicrobials from human skin commensal bacteria protect against *Staphylococcus aureus* and are deficient in atopic dermatitis. *Sci Transl Med*, 9(378): pii: eaah4680.

[166] Myles, I. A., Earland, N. J., Anderson, E. D., Moore, I. N., Kieh, M. D., Williams, K. W., Saleem, A., Fontecilla, N. M., Welch, P. A., Darnell, D. A., Barnhart, L. A., Sun, A. A., Uzel, G., and Datta, S. K. (2018). First-in-human topical microbiome transplantation with *Roseomonas mucosa* for atopic dermatitis. *JCI Insight*, 3(9). pii: 120608.

[167] Richard, G., *Identifier NCT03151148. Targeted microbiome transplant in atopic dermatitis.* Accessed June 22, 2020. Available from: https://www.clinicaltrials.gov/ct2/show/NCT03151148? term=NCT03151148&draw=2&rank=1.

[168] Totte J. E. E., van Doorn, M. B., and Pasmans, S. G. M. A. (2017). Successful treatment of chronic *Staphylococcus aureus*-related dermatoses with the topical endolysin staphefekt SA.100: a report of 3 cases. *Case Rep Dermatol*, 9(2):19-25.

[169] Herpers, B., Badoux, P., Pietersma, F., Eichenseher, F., and Loessner, M (2014). Specific lysis of methicillin susceptible and

resistant *Staphylococcus aureus* by the endolysin Staphefekt SA. 100 ™, *24th European Congress of Clinical Microbiology and Infectious Diseases (ECCMID)*. Abstract.

[170] Totte, J., de Wit, J., Pardo, L., Schuren, F., van Doorn, M., and Pasmans, S. (2017). Targeted anti-staphylococcal therapy with endolysins in atopic dermatitis and the effect on steroid use, disease severity and the microbiome: study protocol for a randomized controlled trial (MAAS trial). *Trials*, 18(1):4.

Biographical Sketch

Ge Peng

Affiliation: Department of Dermatology and Allergology, and Atopy (Allergy) Research Center, Juntendo University Graduate School of Medicine, Tokyo, Japan.

Education:

- Sep 2010 – Jun 2015: Faculty of Medicine, Southern Medical University, Guangzhou, Guangdong, China.
- Sep 2015 – Jun 2018: School of Medicine, China Medical University, Shenyang, Liaoning, China. Master's program, Department of Dermatology and Venereology.
- Oct 2016 – Sep 2017: Graduate School of Medicine, Dentistry and Pharmaceutical Sciences, Okayama University, Okayama, Japan. Research Fellow, Department of Immunology.
- Oct 2018 – Mar 2019: Graduate School of Medicine, Juntendo University, Tokyo, Japan. Research Fellow, Department of Dermatology and Allergology

- Apr 2019 – Present: Graduate School of Medicine, Juntendo University, Tokyo, Japan: PhD program, Department of Dermatology and Allergology

Honors:

1. *Innovation Experiment Award (2013)*: Awarded by the Southern Medical University to the excellent students in Innovation Experiment Competition.
2. *Best Student Award (2014)*: Awarded by the Southern Medical University to the students with outstanding academic profile and excellent manners.
3. *Graduate Student Academic Scholarship, 3rd Prize (2015)*: Awarded by the Southern Medical University to the students with excellent academic profile.
4. *Japan Student Services Organization (JASSO) Scholarship (2016)*: Awarded to the international exchange students with excellent academic profile to study in Japan.
5. *Graduate Student Academic Scholarship, 2nd Prize (2017)*: Awarded by the Graduate School of China Medical University to the students with excellent academic profile.
6. *National Graduate Student Scholarship (2017)*: Awarded by the Ministry of Education of China to students with excellent academic profile.
7. *Graduate Student Academic Scholarship, 1st Prize (2018)*: Awarded by the Graduate School of China Medical University to the students with excellent academic profile.
8. *Honorary Graduate Student Award (2018)*: Awarded by the Ministry of Education of Liaoning Province, China, to the graduate students with excellent academic profile during the master's program.
9. *Monbukagakusho Scholarship (2018)*: Awarded by the Ministry of Education, Culture, Sports, Science, and Technology Japan. It is

one of the most prestigious scholarships offered by the Japanese Government.

10. *Juntendo University Project Research Grant (2019)*: Awarded by Juntendo University Graduate School of Medicine to the Ph.D. students with excellent research project.
11. *LEO Foundation Skin Immunology Research Center Summer School Travel Award (2020)*: Awarded by LEO Foundation Skin Immunology Research Center, University of Copenhagen to the Ph.D. students and postdoctoral fellows to attend a three-day training course on the skin and immunological diseases.
12. *Society for Investigative Dermatology / Japanese Society for Investigative Dermatology Young Fellow Collegiality Award (2020)*: Awarded by the Japanese Society for Investigative Dermatology to the young members to visit international universities.
13. *Juntendo University Project Research Grant (2020)*: Awarded by Juntendo University Graduate School of Medicine to the Ph.D. students with excellent research project.

Publications from the Last 3 Years:

1. Cheng, R., Zhang, H., Zong, W., Tang, J., Han, X., Zhang, L., Zhang, X., Gu, H., Shu, Y., Peng, G., Huang, L., Liu, Q., Gao, X., Guo, Y., and Yao, Z. (2020). Development and validation of new diagnostic criteria for atopic dermatitis in children of China. *J Eur Acad Dermatol Venereol*, 34(3), 542–548. doi: 10.1111/jdv.15979.
2. Wu, W., Peng, G., Yang, F., Zhang, Y., Mu, Z., and Han, X. (2019). Sulforaphane has a therapeutic effect in an atopic dermatitis murine model and activates the Nrf2/HO-1 axis. *Mol Med Rep*, 20(2), 1761–1771. doi: 10.3892/mmr.2019.10405.
3. Peng, G., Mu, Z., Cui, L., Liu, P., Wang, Y., Wu, W., & Han, X. (2018). Anti-IL-33 Antibody has a therapeutic effect in an atopic dermatitis murine model induced by 2, 4-dinitrochlorobenzene. *Inflammation*, 41(1), 154–163. doi: 10.1007/s10753-017-0673-7.

4. Wang, Y., Zhang, Y., Peng, G., and Han, X. (2018). Glycyrrhizin ameliorates atopic dermatitis-like symptoms through inhibition of HMGB1. *Int Immunopharmacol*, 60, 9–17. doi: 10.1016/j.intimp.2018.04.029.
5. Zhang, Y., Peng, G., Wang, Y., Cui, L., Wu, W., Wang, L., Liu, C., and Han, X. (2017). Silencing of astrocyte elevated gene-1 inhibits proliferation and migration of melanoma cells and induces apoptosis. *Clin Exp Pharmacol Physiol*, 44(7), 815–826. doi: 10.1111/1440-1681.12767.

In: Atopic Dermatitis
Editor: Andreas Maur

ISBN: 978-1-53618-520-1

Chapter 5

EVALUATION OF THE CLINICAL RESPONSE OF SOME INTERVENTIONS IN DERMATITIS

Jorge Sanchez*[1,*], *MD, MSc, EAC,
Ana M. Carmona-Gil*[2,3], *MSc
and Juan Maldonado-Estrada*[2], *MSc, PhD
[1]Group of Clinical and Experimental Allergy, IPS Universitaria, University of Antioquia, Medellin, Colombia
[2]OHVRI Group (One Health and Veterinary Innovative Research and Development), School of Veterinary Medicine, Faculty of Agrarian Sciences, University of Antioquia, Medellin, Colombia
[3]Centro de Dermatología Veterinaria (DermaVet), Medellin, Colombia

* Corresponding Author's E-mail: Jorge Sanchez jorgem.sanchez@udea.edu.co.

Abstract

Multiple treatments have been proposed for atopic dermatitis, however not all of them are useful for all people. In this chapter, we review some proposed interventions in the management of atopic dermatitis and the population group that can benefit the most according to the severity of the symptoms, the mechanism of action of the intervention and the possible adverse effects. Dogs share many common characteristics with humans in the pathogenesis of the disease, perhaps due to their mutual coexistence. At the final of the chapter we present a comparison of the therapies used in humans and their usefulness (or not) in pets as part of integrative medicine.

Keywords: allergy, allergen, atopy, dermatitis, eczema, probiotics, antihistamines, dupilumab, microbiota

Introduction

Atopic dermatitis affects a large part of the population, particularly children under 5 years [1-4]. In children, the disease tends to remit during adolescence, however, in 10 to 15% of cases it does not disappear and, on the contrary, it can worsen in adulthood. It usually precedes the development of other allergic diseases such as food allergy, asthma, rhinitis and/or conjunctivitis, so it is considered an important risk factor for these diseases [5, 6].

Atopic dermatitis has a great impact on the quality of life of patients. The frequency of physiological or psychiatric problems in patients with moderate to severe dermatitis is higher than those in patients with diabetes mellitus [7]. The economic cost of skin care and medical treatment has increased in the last years [8-10].

Although there are excellent guidelines that offer an appropriate approach for the management of this disease [11, 12]. Little has been studied about the real impact of different management alternatives. Therefore, even if the current guidelines are based on the best available evidence, an evaluation of this evidence is needed at the time of deciding its applicability, what can be measured better with a systematically revision.

Since each patient must receive personalized treatment, the recommendations presented here may not be appropriate for all patients, but offer a starting point for management based on current scientific evidence.

These recommendations are focused on outpatient clinical management with atopic dermatitis of any age [13]. Management in hospitalization and/or emergencies are not covered in this chapter.

Questions of Interest

In many countries, the term "dermatitis" is used as equivalent to "eczema", so in this guideline and in the bibliographic search we use both as synonyms [14-17]. Chronic eczema, could have different pathogenesis; while confirmatory immunological studies are done terms like "atopy dermatitis" or "allergy eczema" have to be avoided and only used if a mediation IgE or Th2 is demonstrated by diagnostic tests of the disease and "non-atopic eczema" when it is discarded.

In this chapter we review some interventions that could help in the treatment of chronic dermatitis. For each intervention the clinical impact and side effects were evaluated; Conditional recommendations for each intervention were proposed according to patients' characteristics.

Bibliographic Search

We systematically searched articles from 2000 to February 2020 from "Medline" and "LILACs" electronic databases. Articles in English, Spanish and Portuguese were reviewed. More information for bibliographic search is presented in [18].

Studies were included if they provided empirical data related to aim questions (clinical trials, cohort studies, case-control studies). We excluded narrative reviews and case reports. We circulate the bibliography collected among the members of the team; In case any of the staff members consider it was necessary to include an additional reference, this was discussed.

Classification of Atopic Dermatitis in Clinical Practice

Chronic eczema can be classified in several ways [19]. Some proposals of classification according to endotypes have been done [20, 21], but their utility in clinical practice is unclear. The presence of atopy or not seems to be associated with clinical characteristics of the patient and the probability of remission or not, so the classification of allergic or non-allergic eczema according to the result skin prick test or IgE serum can be useful in the clinical practice. Nevertheless, a positive specifics IgE test are not always associated with clinical relevance and additional tests like restriction test or challenge test are required to evaluated the clinical impact.

The classification of the severity is established through the use of different scoring scales, such as: Severity Scoring Atopic Dermatitis (SCORAD) and Eczema Area and Severity Index (EASI). These scores are defined according to three parameters: extension of the disease, type of injury and some scales also includes pruritus and sleep disturbance as perceived by the patient. Each scale have their particular characteristics, but the used of anyone of them improve the evaluation of the clinical severity ant treatment response.

Recommendation

Severity classification scales are available to all physicians and there are useful to define interventions for all patients. Classification according to atopy or not seems to be useful for the prognostic of duration in children.

Prevention of Atopic Dermatitis

Primary prevention is focus in the preclusion of the disease. For atopic dermatitis there is not interventions with high evidence for primary prevention. The increase of sIgA levels with breast milk [22] and the use of milk hydrolyzed formulas in infants with sIgE sensitization reduced the cumulative prevalence of eczema [23]. Although these results are supported by some studies, other investigations do not reproduce these results, so their implementation cannot be widely recommended.

In two multicenter studies it was demonstrated that the daily use of emollients, significantly reduced the cumulative incidence of atopic dermatitis at 12 and 36 months, which corresponded to a relative risk reduction of 30 to 50% [24, 25]. It is necessary to evaluate the cost-effectiveness of this intervention [26].

Secondary prevention is focus in preclusion of higher severity, comorbidities or side effects from treatment interventions. The daily use of emollients in patients with mild-moderate disease prevents and delays exacerbations, as well as decreases the use of topical steroids and prolonged eczema-free time [27-29]. Although there is controversial evidence [30], it seems that vitamin D supplementation reduce severity in some patients [31, 32].

Recommendation

Early skin hydration (first 6 months of life) seems to decrease the risk of dermatitis and control of inflammation, improves the clinical control of dermatitis and avoid severe activity of the disease. These recommendations are applicable to patients from any age and to neonates without dermatitis.

Probiotics in Atopic Dermatitis

Microbial colonization of skin begins start few minutes after birth. It could be different depending of environmental factors like the type of delivery; cesarean delivery children have a cutaneous microbiota profile that resembles maternal skin, while cutaneous microbiota of vaginal delivery children has a more diversified profile, similar to the maternal vaginal scenario [33]. During puberty, new changes occur in skin microbiota [34]. There are several mechanisms by which changes in microbial skin diversity (dysbiosis) affect the development of atopic dermatitis; the production, by these dysbiotic bacteria, of several enzymes, such as: proteases (which induce corneocyte desquamation); lipases (which break down lipids of skin barrier); ceramidases (which break down the ceramides present in the barrier structure) [35, 36]. This bacterial overgrowth, with subsequent biofilm formation, mainly related to the pathogenic strains of *Staphylococcus aureus* (methicillin-resistant *Staphylococcus aureus* (MRSA)), would be directly related to changes in the cutaneous barrier [37-39].

Cutaneous microbiota is associated with dermatitis severity, but it is less clear its effect in the pathogenesis; it would also be expected that antibiotic interventions could improvement the dermatitis symptom scores. However, a systematic review [40], in 21 studies with different intervene-tions (oral antibiotics, antibacterial soaps, topical steroids/antibiotics/ antifungal, baths with antibacterial solutions) did not show statistically significant differences.

Probiotics could help dermatitis through restoration in the function of the intestinal barrier, degrading food antigens, regulating the Th1 and Th2 response, regulating the composition and activity of the intestinal microbiota and stimulating the production of IgA [41]. The WAO (Word Allergy Organization) in a systematic review indicates that is likely net benefit from using probiotics the primary prevention of eczema [42]. The use of *Lactobacillus rhamnosus, Lactobacillus salivarius, Bifidobacterium lactis* and others, in several small studies has shown relief of symptoms that results in an improvement of SCORAD [43, 44], being more effective during the first 2 years of life.

Although probiotics are safe and are used as a reasonable option for preventive treatment of dermatitis in children under 6 months of age or high-risk pregnant women, their impact on active treatment appears to be reduced [45, 46].

However, in order to apply this recommendation, it is necessary to resolve several practical questions that currently do not have an answer: Does the type microbiota affect the impact of probiotics? What dosage? For how long? What strains to use? [47]. The lack of control of these variables in the different clinical trials limits the ability to implement this intervention.

Recommendation

The cutaneous microbiota influences the control of atopic dermatitis. There is a potential effect of the use of probiotics in the prevention of atopic dermatitis, however, methodological limitations, a wide variety of strains and the dosage schemes, lead to discordant and contradictory results and their routine use is not recommended.

Restriction Diet

Frequently, patients associate food consumption with the onset or worsening of disease [48-50]. The sensitization to foods in children with atopic dermatitis is very prevalent (20 to 60%), being the majority of cases asymptomatic (without clinical relevance (50 to 80%)) [51, 52]. The subgroup of moderate to severe atopic dermatitis have a greater risk of sensitization to foods and this is translated into a high risk of true food allergy [51, 53, 54]. The clinical history, along with allergological evaluation, can help to identify suspect foods, but it is necessary to verify with restriction diets for 3 to 4 weeks or controlled oral challenges.

The avoidance of foods previously tolerated or never ingested due to a positive skin test without clinical confirmation of hypersensitivity reactions, is associated with an increased risk of severe reactions, after their reintroduction into the regular diet [55-58]. Therefore, the avoidance of food should only occur in cases of chronic eczema with the confirmation of clinical impact [59]. In cases that negative results in oral challenges or food restrictions did not improve chronic eczema, foods must be reintroduced [60]. Many of the food allergies can be overcome over time, generally preceded by a decrease in IgE but not always; therefore, if the patient achieves good clinical control, the atopic tests can be repeated and, according to the result, consider carrying out a controlled introduction of food.

Recommendation

Only atopy to foods is not enough to initiate a dietary restriction. In patients with an objective demonstration or high suspect of exacerbation of dermatitis by a food, dietary restriction is indicated, nevertheless when atopic dermatitis is controlled it may be possible to consider food reintroduction.

Non-Pharmacological Interventions

The treatment of chronic dermatitis is a challenge because it is a chronic disease, with periods of outbreak and remission. The therapeutic approach of dermatitis includes two aspects: the management of eczematous lesion and the prevention of new exacerbations.

The emollient preparation should be chosen according to the degree of dryness of the skin, the areas of application, and the acceptance by the patient [61, 62]. Use of tight or rough clothes, products for personal use with alcohol or perfume, exposure to heat or activities with inducing heavy sweating among others, should be avoided as far as possible [63, 64]. Some recommendations with low evidence but cost-effective are usually done: The bath should be tempered and brief, no more than 5 minutes. The hygiene of the skin should be smooth, and the scabs should be removed. Avoid perfumes. The use of hypochlorite during bath could reduce colonization of some bacteria [65-67]. The use of comfortable, loose clothing preferably made of cotton seems to prevent skin exacerbation.

Recommendation

The hydration of the skin is a non-pharmacological intervention with adequate evidence for the treatment and prevention of eczema exacerbation in dermatitis. Although the evidence is weak and the magnitude of this measure is not known, we recommend the following basic care:

1. Make short baths of maximum five minutes, with warm or slightly cold water (ideally, twice a day) and avoid the frequent use of soaps.
2. Drying should be done gently and avoid rubbing with rough towels or using dryers.
3. After activities that produce sweating, such as exercise, you should take a new bath; likewise, when exposed to a probable allergen in the patient (pets, pollen grains, etc.).
4. Apply moisturizing creams or lotions at least once a day (intensity varies according to severity).
5. Keep nails short and clean.
6. Avoid irritating products: perfumes, soaps, extreme temperatures, tight clothes, detergent residue on clothes, etc.
7. Exposure to the sun at least 15 minutes a day and, in case of prolonged exposures, use sun bleach.
8. We discourage the use of products with perfume or clothing that may induce an increase in sweating.

Traditional Pharmacological Interventions

Among the most common traditional pharmacological treatments used are oral antihistamines, topical steroids, and topical calcineurin inhibitors.

Topical Steroids

For anti-inflammatory treatment, topical steroids remain the cornerstone in the management of dermatitis [19, 68, 69] Despite the widespread and undeniable usefulness of steroids in dermatitis, there are few controlled studies supporting their uses or how to use them; since patients with dermatitis may require prolonged use of steroid, justifiable concerns about the high risk of local and systemic adverse effects arise.

Different schemes have been proposed in the use of steroids and some common points are present: Steroids with high potency should be used only in patients with moderate to severe atopic dermatitis, and should be avoided in the facial, folds and perennial regions, and they must be used with caution in children under two years. They could be considered in those three areas previously described in exceptional cases and for periods not exceeding 7 days. In all patients they should be used for the minimum possible time and switching to medium or low power steroids according to the control of the patient. The continuous use of steroids for prolonged periods in wide body extensions (even mild steroids) can have similar risk of adverse effects than oral or intravenous steroids. The use of intermittent treatment appears to reduce this risk even with high potency steroids [69].

Steroid use with moisturizer seems to improve the power of the steroid and increase the time of its effect on the skin, so it is recommended their joint application in mixtures or separately, according to the severity of the symptoms. Most oily moisturizers may promote absorption of steroids for its occlusive effect. Proactive management consisting of intermittent application of a low power steroid or calcineurin inhibitors, appears to significantly reduce the risk of relapse in patients under control [61].

The application of steroids more than once a day seems to report no advantage but increases the risk of adverse effects, especially in the sensitive areas of the face or skin folds. In acute injuries, it is advisable to mix the steroid with an emollient to prevent irritation in the area ant to increase absorption. The application of occlusive steroid systems should be performed only by the indication of specialists (allergists or dermatologists) [19, 68].

Calcineurin Inhibitors

There are two topical calcineurin inhibitors: tacrolimus and pimecrolimus. Both have proven efficacy in dermatitis in active and proactive treatment [70, 71]. In practice, they can be used for the same indications as a steroid of medium (tacrolimus 1%) or low power (tacrolimus 0.03%, pimecrolimus 1%), with the advantage that if continuous treatment is required, it will have a lower risk of adverse effects and it will not cause skin atrophy. However, it is necessary to avoid open injuries because they often produce burning feeling. Other less common side effects include eczema herpeticum or molluscum. Although there is no evidence to show a causal relationship between cancer and the use of topical calcineurin inhibitors, it is recommended to be aware of the possible association during follow-up of patients with indication of this treatment for active and proactive management.

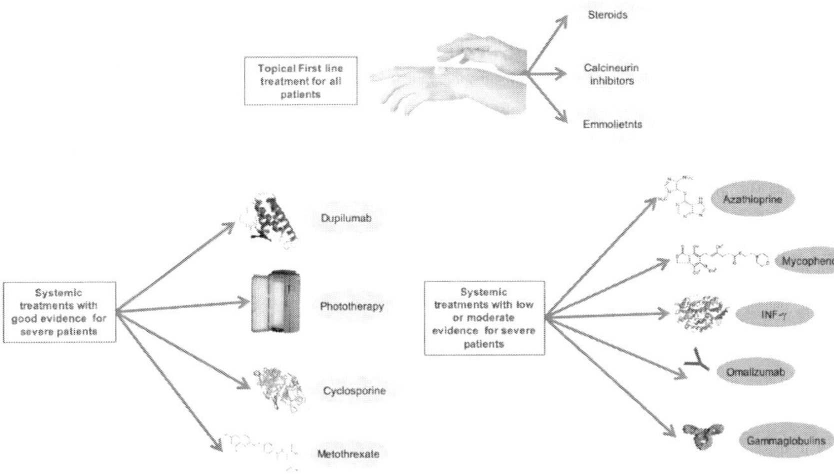

Figure 1. Treatments for atopic dermatitis.
Different treatments have been proposed for atopic dermatitis, we present the topical treatment that is recommended for any patient; systemic treatments with good or moderate/low evidence for severe patients is also presented.

Antihistamines

Pruritus is usually the most distressing feature of dermatitis [72]. Histamine is one of the multiple mediators of itching in dermatitis. However it is not clear if it has a key role [73]. There are no large, randomized, double-blind, and placebo-controlled studies with precise endpoints on the efficacy of antihistamines in atopic dermatitis. Antihistamines (especially first generation) have been used in dermatitis to reduce scratching: nevertheless, in most of the studies are not more effective than placebo [74-77]. Nevertheless, some studies especially with second-generation antihistamines, suggest a possible positive effect in pruritus and repair of the cutaneous tissue [78-81]; these effect increase with a topical steroid [82].

First generation sedating antihistamines have been used in dermatitis to promote sleep [74, 75] but sedating antihistamines reduce the rapid-eye-movement (REM)-sleep, affecting the quality of sleep and interfere directly in work efficiency in adults, and learning skills in children [83].

Recommendation

All patients with atopic dermatitis for active and proactive management have to use topical steroids or calcineurin inhibitors. The power of steroid and frequency of use will depend on the course and severity of patients. The use of antihistamines is more questionable.

New Pharmacological Interventions

Most patients with atopic dermatitis respond satisfactorily to conventional topical management. However, 10 to 50% of patients may not achieve adequate disease control with these regimens and require systemic immunomodulatory/immunosuppressive therapies. Before considering a systemic therapy, it should be determined whether the failure of conventional therapies is due to the severity of the disease, comorbidities or lack of adherence to the treatment. We present some details of each one of some of these therapies. Some of these therapies are not approved yet for dermatitis but there use over-the-counter. It's very common.

Crisaborole

A topical phosphodiesterase 4 (PDE4) inhibitor, became available in late 2016 in the United States and Europe for mild-to-moderate dermatitis. It can be used topically. Clinical trials have demonstrated its efficacy in treating patients with mild to moderate atopic dermatitis (children > 2 years) (NCT02118766; NCT02118792) [84, 85]. The potency of crisaborole seems to be equivalent to that of a steroid of moderate potency, but the frequency of adverse effects seems to be lower; to date there is no evidence of atrophy, telangiectasia or hypopigmentation resulting from its use [86]. However, there are few studies of equivalence or superiority comparing this molecule with topical steroids, so at the moment, crisaborole is recommended at the same level as the use of steroids o calcineurin inhibitors.

Dupilumab

It was approved in early 2017 for moderate-to-severe adult dermatitis [87, 88]. Dupilumab is a fully human monoclonal antibody that blocks the alpha subunit of the receptor interleukin-4 and interleukin-13. The blockade by dupilumab of these key drivers of type 2 helper T-cell (Th2)-mediated inflammation help in the treatment of atopic dermatitis. Patients treated with dupilumab had marked and rapid improvement in all the evaluated measures of atopic dermatitis disease activity and reduces the need for systemic steroids (NCT01259323, NCT01385657, NCT01 639040, and NCT01548404.) [88-91].

Phototherapy or Photochemotherapy

It is one of the alternatives with the highest number of articles and some RCT that support its effectiveness. However, the need for assistance to the center of execution between 2 to 4 times per week limits its access and use [92-95]. Different forms of light therapy are available, and have showed efficacy: narrowband (NB)-UVB, broadband (BB)-UVB, UVA, UVA1, cold-light UVA1, UVA and UVB (UVAB), full-spectrum light (including UVA, infrared and visible light), psoralen plus UVA (PUVA), and other forms of phototherapy. One of the principal limitations for phototherapy is the requirement to attend several times per week for its application. However some new modalities for home application are being developed [96].

Systemic Corticosteroids (SCSs)

There are not recommended as a control intervention for the treatment of dermatitis. Their use should be limited to very short courses (up to 1 week) during acute flares in need of immediate relief and as a transition to steroid-sparing therapies because of the potential for adverse effects [69, 97, 98].

Cyclosporine A (CSA)

It is approved drug for severe dermatitis in some countries and numerous studies showed improvement of the skin symptoms by at least 50% after 6 to 8 weeks of therapy [99-103]. Once the drug is stopped the symptoms reappear quickly, eventually reaching pretreatment values approximately 8 weeks after the end of treatment [101, 103]. CSA has been shown to be effective and relatively safe in adults who received up to 1 year of continuous treatment [104-108], but some of these studies had a high dropout rate [108]. The staff recommended choosing the regimen on an individual basis; it could be reasonable to start with a dose of 2.5 mg/kg/day [106, 109], unless a rapid improvement is considered necessary, when a dose of up to 5 mg/kg/day may be used [108, 110, 111].

Methotrexate (MTX)

Patients receiving MTX should be monitored for hepatic and pulmonary toxicity and myelosuppression [112]. Different studies have shown a good efficacy for MTX [113, 114]. MTX has some advantages and disadvantages compared to CSA but it seems to have a similar effectivity [114-116]; The onset of control seems to be faster with ciclosporin, but relapse after stopping the medication seems to be less frequent with MTX

Azathioprine (AZA)

Efficacy of AZA (2.5 mg/kg/day) was tested in some RCT especially in adults [99, 117], with efficacy (30 to 70%) in the severity of eczema and skin pruritus. In a RCT comparing MTX (10-22.5 mg/wk) with AZA (1.5-2.5 mg/kg/d). At week 12, no statistically significant differences were found in the clinical impact (MTX SCORAD of 42% (SD, 18%) vs AZA 39% (SD, 25%)) [118], but abnormalities in blood count (mostly lymphocytopenia) were statistically significantly more frequent in the AZA group ($P = 0.002$).

Mycophenolate (MMF)

Some case reports or uncontrolled clinical trial data from adults indicate that MMF could be effective in dermatitis [119-123]. In an observer-blinded randomized controlled trial in 55 patients, lower dose CSA (3 mg/kg/d) was found to be equally effective to oral MMF (EC-MPS, 1440 mg/d) as a maintenance therapy for severe dermatitis during a maintenance phase of 30 weeks and a 12-week follow-up period [104]. The MMF group had a slower onset of action with 29% of the MMF patients requiring short courses of systemic glucocorticoids compared with none in the CSA group [124].

Recommendation

Multiple effective measures have been tested in dermatitis which allow adequate control of symptoms when traditional treatments are not enough. Non-pharmacological measures should be used before or in parallel with pharmacological treatment due to their better safety profile and good efficacy.

The decision to start systemic therapy should be based on the severity of the symptoms, but also on the impact on the patient's quality of life, as well as consideration of risks and benefits of systemic therapies for each individual patient.

TRANSLATIONAL MEDICINE FOR VETERINARY APLICATIONS

Animals can have atopic dermatitis. Dogs share many common characteristics with humans in the pathogenesis of the disease, perhaps due to their mutual coexistence and have served as models for human treatments and vice versa [125, 126]. The great relevance of these pets in the life of humans and their similarity in the pathogenesis motivates us to present in Table 1 a comparison of the therapies used in humans and their usefulness (or not) in pets. More information about pathogenesis is presented in the chapter "*Immunopathogenesis of Canine Atopic Dermatitis: comparison to human atopic dermatitis. A Review*".

Table 1. Comparison of therapies for atopic dermatitis in humans and dogs

Intervention	Humans	Dogs
Emollients	High effective	Approved
Topical steroids	High effective	Approved
Calcineurin inhibitors	High effective	Approved
Dupilumab	High effective	Not tested
Phototherapy	Effective	Tested but not approved
Cyclosporine	Effective	Approved
Methotrexate	Effective	Tested but not approved
Azathioprine	Moderate effective	Tested but not approved
Mycophenolate	Moderate effective	Tested but not approved
INF-gamma	Low effective	Not approved
Omalizumab	Low effective	Not approved
Gammaglobulins	Low effective	Tested but not approved

In Orange first line of treatment, blue second line, green third line.

References

[1] Odhiambo JA, Williams HC, Clayton TO, Robertson CF, Asher MI, Group IPTS. Global variations in prevalence of eczema symptoms in children from ISAAC Phase Three. *J Allergy Clin Immunol.* 2009;124(6):1251-8.e23.

[2] Grize L, Gassner M, Wüthrich B, Bringolf-Isler B, Takken-Sahli K, Sennhauser FH, et al. Trends in prevalence of asthma, allergic rhinitis and atopic dermatitis in 5-7-year old Swiss children from 1992 to 2001. *Allergy.* 2006;61(5):556-62.

[3] Weber AS, Haidinger G. The prevalence of atopic dermatitis in children is influenced by their parents' education: results of two

cross-sectional studies conducted in Upper Austria. *Pediatr Allergy Immunol.* 2010;21(7):1028-35.

[4] Solé D, Mallol J, Wandalsen GF, Aguirre V, Group LAIPS. Prevalence of symptoms of eczema in Latin America: results of the International Study of Asthma and Allergies in Childhood (ISAAC) Phase 3. *J Investig Allergol Clin Immunol.* 2010;20(4):311-23.

[5] Barnetson RS, Rogers M. Childhood atopic eczema. *BMJ.* 2002;324(7350):1376-9.

[6] Gustafsson D, Sjöberg O, Foucard T. Development of allergies and asthma in infants and young children with atopic dermatitis--a prospective follow-up to 7 years of age. *Allergy.* 2000;55(3):240-5.

[7] Kemp AS. Cost of illness of atopic dermatitis in children: a societal perspective. *Pharmacoeconomics.* 2003;21(2):105-13.

[8] Lapidus CS, Schwarz DF, Honig PJ. Atopic dermatitis in children: who cares? Who pays? *J Am Acad Dermatol.* 1993;28(5 Pt 1):699-703.

[9] Lawson V, Lewis-Jones MS, Finlay AY, Reid P, Owens RG. The family impact of childhood atopic dermatitis: the Dermatitis Family Impact Questionnaire. *Br J Dermatol.* 1998;138(1):107-13.

[10] Adamson AS. The Economics Burden of Atopic Dermatitis. *Adv Exp Med Biol.* 2017;1027:79-92.

[11] Wollenberg A, Barbarot S, Bieber T, Christen-Zaech S, Deleuran M, Fink-Wagner A, et al. Consensus-based European guidelines for treatment of atopic eczema (atopic dermatitis) in adults and children: part I. *J Eur Acad Dermatol Venereol.* 2018;32(5):657-82.

[12] Wollenberg A, Barbarot S, Bieber T, Christen-Zaech S, Deleuran M, Fink-Wagner A, et al. Consensus-based European guidelines for treatment of atopic eczema (atopic dermatitis) in adults and children: part II. *J Eur Acad Dermatol Venereol.* 2018;32(6):850-78.

[13] Davies E, Rogers NK, Lloyd-Lavery A, Grindlay DJC, Thomas KS. What's new in atopic eczema? An analysis of systematic reviews published in 2015. Part 1: epidemiology and methodology. *Clin Exp Dermatol.* 2018;43(4):375-9.

[14] Schäfer T, Krämer U, Vieluf D, Abeck D, Behrendt H, Ring J. The excess of atopic eczema in East Germany is related to the intrinsic type. *Br J Dermatol.* 2000;143(5):992-8.

[15] Böhme M, Wickman M, Lennart Nordvall S, Svartengren M, Wahlgren CF. Family history and risk of atopic dermatitis in children up to 4 years. *Clin Exp Allergy.* 2003;33(9):1226-31.

[16] Schmid-Grendelmeier P, Flückiger S, Disch R, Trautmann A, Wüthrich B, Blaser K, et al. IgE-mediated and T cell-mediated autoimmunity against manganese superoxide dismutase in atopic dermatitis. *J Allergy Clin Immunol.* 2005;115(5):1068-75.

[17] Johansson SG, Bieber T, Dahl R, Friedmann PS, Lanier BQ, Lockey RF, et al. Revised nomenclature for allergy for global use: Report of the Nomenclature Review Committee of the World Allergy Organization, October 2003. *J Allergy Clin Immunol.* 2004;113(5): 832-6.

[18] Sánchez J, Sánchez M, Macías-Weinmann A, Barreto B, Ensina L, Uriarte-Obando S, et al. Systematic review about 10 interventions in dermatitis. A document from the Latin American Society of Allergy, Asthma, and Immunology. *Revista Alergia Mexico.* 2019;66(4):426-55

[19] Sánchez J, Páez B, Macías A, Olmos C, de Falco A. Atopic dermatitis guideline. Position paper from the Latin American Society of Allergy, Asthma and Immunology. *Rev Alerg Mex.* 2014; 61(3):178-211.

[20] Thijs JL, Strickland I, Bruijnzeel-Koomen CAFM, Nierkens S, Giovannone B, Csomor E, et al. Moving toward endotypes in atopic dermatitis: Identification of patient clusters based on serum biomarker analysis. *J Allergy Clin Immunol.* 2017;140(3):730-7.

[21] Muraro A, Lemanske RF, Hellings PW, Akdis CA, Bieber T, Casale TB, et al. Precision medicine in patients with allergic diseases: Airway diseases and atopic dermatitis-PRACTALL document of the European Academy of Allergy and Clinical Immunology and the American Academy of Allergy, Asthma & Immunology. *J Allergy Clin Immunol.* 2016;137(5):1347-58.

[22] Orivuori L, Mustonen K, Roduit C, Braun-Fahrländer C, Dalphin JC, Genuneit J, et al. Immunoglobulin A and immunoglobulin G antibodies against β-lactoglobulin and gliadin at age 1 associate with immunoglobulin E sensitization at age 6. *Pediatr Allergy Immunol.* 2014;25(4):329-37.

[23] von Berg A, Filipiak-Pittroff B, Schulz H, Hoffmann U, Link E, Sußmann M, et al. Allergic manifestation 15 years after early intervention with hydrolyzed formulas--the GINI Study. *Allergy.* 2016;71(2):210-9.

[24] Simpson EL, Chalmers JR, Hanifin JM, Thomas KS, Cork MJ, McLean WH, et al. Emollient enhancement of the skin barrier from birth offers effective atopic dermatitis prevention. *J Allergy Clin Immunol.* 2014;134(4):818-23.

[25] Horimukai K, Morita K, Narita M, Kondo M, Kitazawa H, Nozaki M, et al. Application of moisturizer to neonates prevents development of atopic dermatitis. *J Allergy Clin Immunol.* 2014;134(4):824-30.e6.

[26] Chalmers JR, Haines RH, Mitchell EJ, Thomas KS, Brown SJ, Ridd M, et al. Effectiveness and cost-effectiveness of daily all-over-body application of emollient during the first year of life for preventing atopic eczema in high-risk children (The BEEP trial): protocol for a randomised controlled trial. *Trials.* 2017;18(1):343.

[27] Tiplica GS, Kaszuba A, Malinauskienė L, Konno P, Boralevi F, Garrigue E, et al. Prevention of Flares in Children with Atopic Dermatitis with Regular Use of an Emollient Containing Glycerol and Paraffin: A Randomized Controlled Study. *Pediatr Dermatol.* 2017;34(3):282-9.

[28] Åkerström U, Reitamo S, Langeland T, Berg M, Rustad L, Korhonen L, et al. Comparison of Moisturizing Creams for the Prevention of Atopic Dermatitis Relapse: A Randomized Double-blind Controlled Multicentre Clinical Trial. *Acta Derm Venereol.* 2015;95(5):587-92.

[29] Fukuie T, Hirakawa S, Narita M, Nomura I, Matsumoto K, Tokura Y, et al. Potential preventive effects of proactive therapy on sensitization in moderate to severe childhood atopic dermatitis: A

randomized, investigator-blinded, controlled study. *J Dermatol.* 2016;43(11):1283-92.

[30] Muehleisen B, Gallo RL. Vitamin D in allergic disease: shedding light on a complex problem. *J Allergy Clin Immunol.* 2013;131(2):324-9.

[31] Camargo CA, Ganmaa D, Sidbury R, Erdenedelger K, Radnaakhand N, Khandsuren B. Randomized trial of vitamin D supplementation for winter-related atopic dermatitis in children. *J Allergy Clin Immunol.* 2014;134(4):831-5.e1.

[32] Sidbury R, Sullivan AF, Thadhani RI, Camargo CA. Randomized controlled trial of vitamin D supplementation for winter-related atopic dermatitis in Boston: a pilot study. *Br J Dermatol.* 2008;159(1):245-7.

[33] Dominguez-Bello MG, Costello EK, Contreras M, Magris M, Hidalgo G, Fierer N, et al. Delivery mode shapes the acquisition and structure of the initial microbiota across multiple body habitats in newborns. *Proc Natl Acad Sci U S A.* 2010;107(26):11971-5.

[34] Park YJ, Lee HK. The Role of Skin and Orogenital Microbiota in Protective Immunity and Chronic Immune-Mediated Inflammatory Disease. *Front Immunol.* 2017;8:1955.

[35] Baldwin HE, Bhatia ND, Friedman A, Eng RM, Seite S. The Role of Cutaneous Microbiota Harmony in Maintaining a Functional Skin Barrier. *J Drugs Dermatol.* 2017;16(1):12-8.

[36] Nakatsuji T, Chen TH, Narala S, Chun KA, Two AM, Yun T, et al. Antimicrobials from human skin commensal bacteria protect against. *Sci Transl Med.* 2017;9(378).

[37] Di Domenico EG, Cavallo I, Bordignon V, Prignano G, Sperduti I, Gurtner A, et al. Inflammatory cytokines and biofilm production sustain *Staphylococcus aureus* outgrowth and persistence: a pivotal interplay in the pathogenesis of Atopic Dermatitis. *Sci Rep.* 2018;8(1):9573.

[38] Jinnestål CL, Belfrage E, Bäck O, Schmidtchen A, Sonesson A. Skin barrier impairment correlates with cutaneous *Staphylococcus aureus* colonization and sensitization to skin-associated microbial antigens

in adult patients with atopic dermatitis. *Int J Dermatol.* 2014;53(1):27-33.

[39] Cavalcante FS, Abad ED, Lyra YC, Saintive SB, Ribeiro M, Ferreira DC, et al. High prevalence of methicillin resistance and PVL genes among *Staphylococcus aureus* isolates from the nares and skin lesions of pediatric patients with atopic dermatitis. *Braz J Med Biol Res.* 2015;48(7):588-94.

[40] Birnie AJ, Bath-Hextall FJ, Ravenscroft JC, Williams HC. Interventions to reduce *Staphylococcus aureus* in the management of atopic eczema. *Cochrane Database Syst Rev.* 2008(3):CD003871.

[41] Yeşilova Y, Çalka Ö, Akdeniz N, Berktaş M. Effect of probiotics on the treatment of children with atopic dermatitis. *Ann Dermatol.* 2012;24(2):189-93.

[42] Fiocchi A, Pawankar R, Cuello-Garcia C, Ahn K, Al-Hammadi S, Agarwal A, et al. World Allergy Organization-McMaster University Guidelines for Allergic Disease Prevention (GLAD-P): Probiotics. *World Allergy Organ J.* 2015;8(1):4.

[43] Niccoli AA, Artesi AL, Candio F, Ceccarelli S, Cozzali R, Ferraro L, et al. Preliminary results on clinical effects of probiotic Lactobacillus salivarius LS01 in children affected by atopic dermatitis. *J Clin Gastroenterol.* 2014;48 Suppl 1:S34-6.

[44] Huang R, Ning H, Shen M, Li J, Zhang J, Chen X. Probiotics for the Treatment of Atopic Dermatitis in Children: A Systematic Review and Meta-Analysis of Randomized Controlled Trials. *Front Cell Infect Microbiol.* 2017;7:392.

[45] Wickens K, Barthow C, Mitchell EA, Stanley TV, Purdie G, Rowden J, et al. Maternal supplementation alone with Lactobacillus rhamnosus HN001 during pregnancy and breastfeeding does not reduce infant eczema. *Pediatr Allergy Immunol.* 2018;29(3):296-302.

[46] Boyle RJ, Bath-Hextall FJ, Leonardi-Bee J, Murrell DF, Tang ML. Probiotics for treating eczema. *Cochrane Database Syst Rev.* 2008(4):CD006135.

[47] Yang HJ, Min TK, Lee HW, Pyun BY. Efficacy of Probiotic Therapy on Atopic Dermatitis in Children: A Randomized, Double-blind, Placebo-controlled Trial. *Allergy Asthma Immunol Res.* 2014;6(3):208-15.

[48] Sánchez J, Sánchez A. Epidemiology of food allergy in Latin America. *Allergol Immunopathol (Madr).* 2015;43(2):185-95.

[49] Sánchez J, Sánchez A. Epidemiologic studies about food allergy and food sensitization in tropical countries. Results and limitations. *Allergol Immunopathol (Madr).* 2019.

[50] Estrada-Reyes E, Pardo-Castañeda MG, Toledo-Bahena ME, Lerma-Ortiz ML, del Río-Navarro B, Nava-Ocampo AA. A case-control study of food hyper-sensitivity, timing of weaning and family history of allergies in young children with atopic dermatitis. *Allergol Immunopathol (Madr).* 2007;35(3):101-4.

[51] Jøhnke H, Norberg LA, Vach W, Høst A, Andersen KE. Patterns of sensitization in infants and its relation to atopic dermatitis. *Pediatr Allergy Immunol.* 2006;17(8):591-600.

[52] Roerdink EM, Flokstra-de Blok BM, Blok JL, Schuttelaar ML, Niggemann B, Werfel T, et al. Association of food allergy and atopic dermatitis exacerbations. *Ann Allergy Asthma Immunol.* 2016; 116(4):334-8.

[53] Rennick GJ, Moore E, Orchard DC. Skin prick testing to food allergens in breast-fed young infants with moderate to severe atopic dermatitis. *Australas J Dermatol.* 2006;47(1):41-5.

[54] Levy SA, Dortas Junior SD, Pires AH, Abe AT, Valle SO, Coelho VP, et al. Atopy patch test (APT) in the diagnosis of food allergy in children with atopic dermatitis. *An Bras Dermatol.* 2012;87(5): 724-8.

[55] David TJ. Anaphylactic shock during elimination diets for severe atopic eczema. *Arch Dis Child.* 1984;59(10):983-6.

[56] Barbi E, Gerarduzzi T, Longo G, Ventura A. Fatal allergy as a possible consequence of long-term elimination diet. *Allergy.* 2004;59(6):668-9.

[57] Flinterman AE, Knulst AC, Meijer Y, Bruijnzeel-Koomen CA, Pasmans SG. Acute allergic reactions in children with AEDS after prolonged cow's milk elimination diets. *Allergy.* 2006;61(3):370-4.

[58] Chang A, Robison R, Cai M, Singh AM. Natural History of Food-Triggered Atopic Dermatitis and Development of Immediate Reactions in Children. *J Allergy Clin Immunol Pract.* 2016;4(2):229-36.e1.

[59] Fleischer DM, Bock SA, Spears GC, Wilson CG, Miyazawa NK, Gleason MC, et al. Oral food challenges in children with a diagnosis of food allergy. *J Pediatr.* 2011;158(4):578-83.e1.

[60] Eapen AA, Kloepfer KM, Leickly FE, Slaven JE, Vitalpur G. Oral food challenge failures among foods restricted because of atopic dermatitis. *Ann Allergy Asthma Immunol.* 2019;122(2):193-7.

[61] Santer M, Rumsby K, Ridd MJ, Francis NA, Stuart B, Chorozoglou M, et al. Adding emollient bath additives to standard eczema management for children with eczema: the BATHE RCT. *Health Technol Assess.* 2018;22(57):1-116.

[62] Antonijević MD, Novac O, O'Hagan BM. Can emollients of similar composition be assumed to be therapeutically equivalent: a comparison of skin occlusivity and emulsion microstructure. *Clin Cosmet Investig Dermatol.* 2018;11:461-5.

[63] Jung HJ, Bae JY, Kim JE, Na CH, Park GH, Bae YI, et al. Survey of disease awareness, treatment behavior and treatment satisfaction in patients with atopic dermatitis in Korea: A multicenter study. *J Dermatol.* 2018;45(10):1172-80.

[64] Sala-Cunill A, Lazaro M, Herráez L, Quiñones MD, Moro-Moro M, Sanchez I, et al. Basic Skin Care and Topical Therapies for Atopic Dermatitis: Essential Approaches and Beyond. *J Investig Allergol Clin Immunol.* 2018;28(6):379-91.

[65] Eriksson S, van der Plas MJA, Mörgelin M, Sonesson A. Antibacterial and antibiofilm effects of sodium hypochlorite against *Staphylococcus aureus* isolates derived from patients with atopic dermatitis. *Br J Dermatol.* 2017;177(2):513-21.

[66] Harris V, Smith SD. Lifting the biofilm lid on the antibacterial and antibiofilm effects of sodium hypochlorite against *Staphylococcus aureus* in atopic dermatitis. *Br J Dermatol.* 2017;177(2):347-8.

[67] Asch S, Vork DL, Joseph J, Major-Elechi B, Tollefson MM. Comparison of bleach, acetic acid, and other topical anti-infective treatments in pediatric atopic dermatitis: A retrospective cohort study on antibiotic exposure. *Pediatr Dermatol.* 2019;36(1):115-20.

[68] Sánchez J, Páez B, Macías-Weinmann A, De Falco A. [Key points for the management of dermatitis in Latin America. The SLAAI Consensus]. *Rev Alerg Mex.* 2015;62(3):226-33.

[69] Yu SH, Drucker AM, Lebwohl M, Silverberg JI. A systematic review of the safety and efficacy of systemic corticosteroids in atopic dermatitis. *J Am Acad Dermatol.* 2018;78(4):733-40.e11.

[70] Siegfried EC, Jaworski JC, Kaiser JD, Hebert AA. Systematic review of published trials: long-term safety of topical corticosteroids and topical calcineurin inhibitors in pediatric patients with atopic dermatitis. *BMC Pediatr.* 2016;16:75.

[71] Beriat GK, Akmansu SH, Doğan C, Taştan E, Topal F, Sabuncuoğlu B. Is pimecrolimus cream (1%) an appropriate therapeutic agent for the treatment of external ear atopic dermatitis? *Med Sci Monit.* 2012;18(4):BR135-43.

[72] Church MK, Maurer M. H1 -Antihistamines and itch in atopic dermatitis. *Exp Dermatol.* 2015;24(5):332-3.

[73] Ohsawa Y, Hirasawa N. The role of histamine H1 and H4 receptors in atopic dermatitis: from basic research to clinical study. *Allergol Int.* 2014;63(4):533-42.

[74] Munday J, Bloomfield R, Goldman M, Robey H, Kitowska GJ, Gwiezdziski Z, et al. Chlorpheniramine is no more effective than placebo in relieving the symptoms of childhood atopic dermatitis with a nocturnal itching and scratching component. *Dermatology.* 2002;205(1):40-5.

[75] Wahlgren CF, Hägermark O, Bergström R. The antipruritic effect of a sedative and a non-sedative antihistamine in atopic dermatitis. *Br J Dermatol.* 1990;122(4):545-51.

[76] Frosch PJ, Schwanitz HJ, Macher E. A double blind trial of H1 and H2 receptor antagonists in the treatment of atopic dermatitis. *Arch Dermatol Res.* 1984;276(1):36-40.

[77] Savin JA, Dow R, Harlow BJ, Massey H, Yee KF. The effect of a new non-sedative H1-receptor antagonist (LN2974) on the itching and scratching of patients with atopic eczema. *Clin Exp Dermatol.* 1986;11(6):600-2.

[78] Hannuksela M, Kalimo K, Lammintausta K, Mattila T, Turjanmaa K, Varjonen E, et al. Dose ranging study: cetirizine in the treatment of atopic dermatitis in adults. *Ann Allergy.* 1993;70(2):127-33.

[79] Langeland T, Fagertun HE, Larsen S. Therapeutic effect of loratadine on pruritus in patients with atopic dermatitis. A multi-crossover-designed study. *Allergy.* 1994;49(1):22-6.

[80] La Rosa M, Ranno C, Musarra I, Guglielmo F, Corrias A, Bellanti JA. Double-blind study of cetirizine in atopic eczema in children. *Ann Allergy.* 1994;73(2):117-22.

[81] Yamanaka K, Motomura E, Noro Y, Umeda K, Morikawa T, Umeda-Togami K, et al. Olopatadine, a non-sedating H1 antihistamine, decreases the nocturnal scratching without affecting sleep quality in atopic dermatitis. *Exp Dermatol.* 2015;24(3):227-9.

[82] Kawashima M, Tango T, Noguchi T, Inagi M, Nakagawa H, Harada S. Addition of fexofenadine to a topical corticosteroid reduces the pruritus associated with atopic dermatitis in a 1-week randomized, multicentre, double-blind, placebo-controlled, parallel-group study. *Br J Dermatol.* 2003;148(6):1212-21.

[83] Church MK, Maurer M, Simons FE, Bindslev-Jensen C, van Cauwenberge P, Bousquet J, et al. Risk of first-generation H(1)-antihistamines: a GA(2)LEN position paper. *Allergy.* 2010;65(4): 459-66.

[84] Paller AS, Tom WL, Lebwohl MG, Blumenthal RL, Boguniewicz M, Call RS, et al. Efficacy and safety of crisaborole ointment, a novel, nonsteroidal phosphodiesterase 4 (PDE4) inhibitor for the topical treatment of atopic dermatitis (AD) in children and adults. *J Am Acad Dermatol.* 2016;75(3):494-503.e6.

[85] Draelos ZD, Stein Gold LF, Murrell DF, Hughes MH, Zane LT. Post Hoc Analyses of the Effect of Crisaborole Topical Ointment, 2% on Atopic Dermatitis: Associated Pruritus from Phase 1 and 2 Clinical Studies. *J Drugs Dermatol.* 2016;15(2):172-6.

[86] Zane LT, Hughes MH, Shakib S. Tolerability of Crisaborole Ointment for Application on Sensitive Skin Areas: A Randomized, Double-Blind, Vehicle-Controlled Study in Healthy Volunteers. *Am J Clin Dermatol.* 2016;17(5):519-26.

[87] Hamilton JD, Suárez-Fariñas M, Dhingra N, Cardinale I, Li X, Kostic A, et al. Dupilumab improves the molecular signature in skin of patients with moderate-to-severe atopic dermatitis. *J Allergy Clin Immunol.* 2014;134(6):1293-300.

[88] Beck LA, Thaçi D, Hamilton JD, Graham NM, Bieber T, Rocklin R, et al. Dupilumab treatment in adults with moderate-to-severe atopic dermatitis. N Engl J Med. 2014;371(2):130-9.

[89] Silverberg JI, Simpson EL, Ardeleanu M, Thaçi D, Barbarot S, Bagel J, et al. Dupilumab provides important clinical benefits to patients with atopic dermatitis who do not achieve clear or almost clear skin according to the Investigator's Global Assessment: a pooled analysis of data from 2 phase III trials. *Br J Dermatol.* 2019.

[90] Storan ER, Woolf RT, Smith CH, Pink A. Clearance of molluscum contagiosum virus infection in patients with atopic eczema treated with dupilumab. *Br J Dermatol.* 2019.

[91] Blauvelt A, Rosmarin D, Bieber T, Simpson EL, Bagel J, Worm M, et al. Improvement of atopic dermatitis with dupilumab occurs equally well across different anatomic regions: data from phase 3 clinical trials. *Br J Dermatol.* 2019.

[92] Tintle S, Shemer A, Suárez-Fariñas M, Fujita H, Gilleaudeau P, Sullivan-Whalen M, et al. Reversal of atopic dermatitis with narrow-band UVB phototherapy and biomarkers for therapeutic response. *J Allergy Clin Immunol.* 2011;128(3):583-93.e1-4.

[93] Clayton TH, Clark SM, Turner D, Goulden V. The treatment of severe atopic dermatitis in childhood with narrowband ultraviolet B phototherapy. *Clin Exp Dermatol.* 2007;32(1):28-33.

[94] Meduri NB, Vandergriff T, Rasmussen H, Jacobe H. Phototherapy in the management of atopic dermatitis: a systematic review. *Photodermatol Photoimmunol Photomed.* 2007;23(4):106-12.

[95] Brownell J, Wang S, Tsoukas MM. Compliance and phototherapy. *Clin Dermatol.* 2016;34(5):582-6.

[96] Cline A, Unrue EL, Collins A, Feldman SR. Adherence to a novel home phototherapy system with integrated features. *Dermatol Online J.* 2019;25(3).

[97] Drucker AM, Eyerich K, de Bruin-Weller MS, Thyssen JP, Spuls PI, Irvine AD, et al. Use of systemic corticosteroids for atopic dermatitis: International Eczema Council consensus statement. *Br J Dermatol.* 2018;178(3):768-75.

[98] Roekevisch E, Spuls PI, Kuester D, Limpens J, Schmitt J. Efficacy and safety of systemic treatments for moderate-to-severe atopic dermatitis: a systematic review. *J Allergy Clin Immunol.* 2014;133(2):429-38.

[99] Berth-Jones J, Takwale A, Tan E, Barclay G, Agarwal S, Ahmed I, et al. Azathioprine in severe adult atopic dermatitis: a double-blind, placebo-controlled, crossover trial. *Br J Dermatol.* 2002;147(2):324-30.

[100] Berth-Jones J, Graham-Brown RA, Marks R, Camp RD, English JS, Freeman K, et al. Long-term efficacy and safety of cyclosporin in severe adult atopic dermatitis. *Br J Dermatol.* 1997;136(1):76-81.

[101] Salek MS, Finlay AY, Luscombe DK, Allen BR, Berth-Jones J, Camp RD, et al. Cyclosporin greatly improves the quality of life of adults with severe atopic dermatitis. A randomized, double-blind, placebo-controlled trial. *Br J Dermatol.* 1993;129(4):422-30.

[102] van Joost T, Heule F, Korstanje M, van den Broek MJ, Stenveld HJ, van Vloten WA. Cyclosporin in atopic dermatitis: a multicentre placebo-controlled study. *Br J Dermatol.* 1994;130(5):634-40.

[103] Sowden JM, Berth-Jones J, Ross JS, Motley RJ, Marks R, Finlay AY, et al. Double-blind, controlled, crossover study of cyclosporin in adults with severe refractory atopic dermatitis. *Lancet.* 1991;338(8760):137-40.

[104] Haeck IM, Knol MJ, Ten Berge O, van Velsen SG, de Bruin-Weller MS, Bruijnzeel-Koomen CA. Enteric-coated mycophenolate sodium versus cyclosporin A as long-term treatment in adult patients with severe atopic dermatitis: a randomized controlled trial. *J Am Acad Dermatol.* 2011;64(6):1074-84.

[105] Koppelhus U, Poulsen J, Grunnet N, Deleuran MS, Obitz E. Cyclosporine and Extracorporeal Photopheresis are Equipotent in Treating Severe Atopic Dermatitis: A Randomized Cross-Over Study Comparing Two Efficient Treatment Modalities. *Front Med (Lausanne).* 2014;1:33.

[106] Zonneveld IM, De Rie MA, Beljaards RC, Van Der Rhee HJ, Wuite J, Zeegelaar J, et al. The long-term safety and efficacy of cyclosporin in severe refractory atopic dermatitis: a comparison of two dosage regimens. *Br J Dermatol.* 1996;135 Suppl 48:15-20.

[107] Granlund H, Erkko P, Remitz A, Langeland T, Helsing P, Nuutinen M, et al. Comparison of cyclosporin and UVAB phototherapy for intermittent one-year treatment of atopic dermatitis. *Acta Derm Venereol.* 2001;81(1):22-7.

[108] Harper JI, Ahmed I, Barclay G, Lacour M, Hoeger P, Cork MJ, et al. Cyclosporin for severe childhood atopic dermatitis: short course versus continuous therapy. *Br J Dermatol.* 2000;142(1):52-8.

[109] Czech W, Bräutigam M, Weidinger G, Schöpf E. A body-weight-independent dosing regimen of cyclosporine microemulsion is effective in severe atopic dermatitis and improves the quality of life. *J Am Acad Dermatol.* 2000;42(4):653-9.

[110] Bunikowski R, Gerhold K, Bräutigam M, Hamelmann E, Renz H, Wahn U. Effect of low-dose cyclosporin a microemulsion on disease severity, interleukin-6, interleukin-8 and tumor necrosis factor alpha production in severe pediatric atopic dermatitis. *Int Arch Allergy Immunol.* 2001;125(4):344-8.

[111] Bunikowski R, Staab D, Kussebi F, Bräutigam M, Weidinger G, Renz H, et al. Low-dose cyclosporin A microemulsion in children with severe atopic dermatitis: clinical and immunological effects. *Pediatr Allergy Immunol.* 2001;12(4):216-23.

[112] Totri CR, Eichenfield LF, Logan K, Proudfoot L, Schmitt J, Lara-Corrales I, et al. Prescribing practices for systemic agents in the treatment of severe pediatric atopic dermatitis in the US and Canada: The PeDRA TREAT survey. *J Am Acad Dermatol.* 2017;76(2):281-5.

[113] Weatherhead SC, Wahie S, Reynolds NJ, Meggitt SJ. An open-label, dose-ranging study of methotrexate for moderate-to-severe adult atopic eczema. *Br J Dermatol.* 2007;156(2):346-51.

[114] Goujon C, Viguier M, Staumont-Sallé D, Bernier C, Guillet G, Lahfa M, et al. Methotrexate Versus Cyclosporine in Adults with Moderate-to-Severe Atopic Dermatitis: A Phase III Randomized Noninferiority Trial. *J Allergy Clin Immunol Pract.* 2018;6(2):562-9.e3.

[115] Law Ping Man S, Bouzillé G, Beneton N, Safa G, Dupuy A, Droitcourt C. Drug survival and postdrug survival of first-line immunosuppressive treatments for atopic dermatitis: comparison between methotrexate and cyclosporine. *J Eur Acad Dermatol Venereol.* 2018.

[116] El-Khalawany MA, Hassan H, Shaaban D, Ghonaim N, Eassa B. Methotrexate versus cyclosporine in the treatment of severe atopic dermatitis in children: a multicenter experience from Egypt. *Eur J Pediatr.* 2013;172(3):351-6.

[117] Meggitt SJ, Gray JC, Reynolds NJ. Azathioprine dosed by thiopurine methyltransferase activity for moderate-to-severe atopic eczema: a double-blind, randomised controlled trial. *Lancet.* 2006;367(9513): 839-46.

[118] Schram ME, Roekevisch E, Leeflang MM, Bos JD, Schmitt J, Spuls PI. A randomized trial of methotrexate versus azathioprine for severe atopic eczema. *J Allergy Clin Immunol.* 2011;128(2):353-9.

[119] Ballester I, Silvestre JF, Pérez-Crespo M, Lucas A. [Severe adult atopic dermatitis: treatment with mycophenolate mofetil in 8 patients]. *Actas Dermosifiliogr.* 2009;100(10):883-7.

[120] Fallah Arani S, Waalboer Spuij R, Nijsten T, Neumann HA, Thio B. Enteric-coated mycophenolate sodium in psoriasis vulgaris: an open pilot study. *J Dermatolog Treat.* 2014;25(1):46-9.

[121] Grundmann-Kollmann M, Podda M, Ochsendorf F, Boehncke WH, Kaufmann R, Zollner TM. Mycophenolate mofetil is effective in the treatment of atopic dermatitis. *Arch Dermatol.* 2001;137(7):870-3.

[122] Murray ML, Cohen JB. Mycophenolate mofetil therapy for moderate to severe atopic dermatitis. *Clin Exp Dermatol.* 2007;32(1):23-7.

[123] Dias-Polak D, Bergman R, Avitan-Hersh E. Mycophenolate mofetil therapy in adult patients with recalcitrant atopic dermatitis. *J Dermatolog Treat.* 2018:1-3.

[124] Heller M, Shin HT, Orlow SJ, Schaffer JV. Mycophenolate mofetil for severe childhood atopic dermatitis: experience in 14 patients. *Br J Dermatol.* 2007;157(1):127-32.

[125] Gortel K. An embarrassment of riches: An update on the symptomatic treatment of canine atopic dermatitis. *Can Vet J.* 2018;59(9):1013-6.

[126] Olivry T, DeBoer D, Favrot C, Jackson H, Mueller R, Nuttall T, et al. Treatment of canine atopic dermatitis: 2010 clinical practice guidelines from the International Task Force on Canine Atopic Dermatitis. *Veterinary Dermatology* 2010;21(3):2233-48.

Reviewed by: Leidy Alvarez MD, MSc. leidyalvarez01@gmail.com; Elizabeth Garcia MD, EAC: eligarcia.gomez@gmail.com

In: Atopic Dermatitis
Editor: Andreas Maur

ISBN: 978-1-53618-520-1

Chapter 6

TRADITIONAL CHINESE MEDICINE AND ATOPIC DERMATITIS – RESEARCH PROMISES

Ben Chung Lap Chan[1,*], Elaine Wat[1], Ellis Kam Lun Hon[1,2], Xiaoxiao Wu[1], Miranda Sin Man Tsang[1], William Cheng[1], Wing Sum Siu[1], Chi Man Koon[1], Jiawei Ling[1], Wenyi Wang[3], Chi Wai Kan[3], Patrick Hui[3], Frency Ng[3], Clara Bik San Lau[1], Chun Kwok Wong[1,4] and Ping Chung Leung[1]

[1]Institute of Chinese Medicine and State Key Laboratory of Research on Bioactivities and Clinical Applications of Medicinal Plants, The Chinese University of Hong Kong, Hong Kong

[2]The Hong Kong Children's Hospital, Hong Kong

[*] Corresponding Author's E-mail: benchan99@cuhk.edu.hk.

[3]Institute of Textiles and Clothing,
The Hong Kong Polytechnic University,
Hung Hom, Kowloon, Hong Kong
[4] Department of Chemical Pathology, The Chinese University of Hong Kong, Hong Kong

ABSTRACT

Being considered as the first step in the "atopic march," atopic dermatitis (AD) may progressively develop from a typical sequence of AD, food allergy, allergic rhinitis and asthma. Patients with AD may need to go through great lengths in order to achieve some relief, while others may even be at the expense of their long-term health. Continuous efforts have been, and are still being made in the search for alternative or adjunct therapies for relieve or treatment. Traditional Chinese Medicine (TCM) has a long history for use in allergies and AD. TCM utilizes herbs that are combined in a prescription in accordance to Chinese medicine theories. With the increasing demand for TCM in recent decades, its efficacy and safety have been frequently questioned. Pentaherbs Formula (PHF) is a Chinese herbal oral concoction modified from an ancient TCM formulation. Previous clinical trials demonstrated its potential in children with moderate-to-severe AD. *In vitro* and *in vivo* experiments further confirmed its efficacy and provided insight on the underlying mechanisms which contribute to the observed beneficial effects. The promises of PHF on AD both clinically and pre-clinically have led to the further exploration of its potential as topical therapy from simple topical lotions, to encapsulation with hydrogel conjugation or even application onto the natural fabric as textile-based transdermal therapy. This chapter will utilize PHF as an example, to illustrate to readers on efforts and stages taken in TCM research in an attempt to adopt this historic and yet unique complementary medicine to become a safer and scientific-based therapy for wider applications.

Keywords: atopic dermatitis, traditional Chinese medicine, pentaherbs, Moutan Cortex, hydrogel, textile

INTRODUCTION

Atopic dermatitis (AD) is a complex disease commonly associated with allergy characterized by various degrees of skin inflammation, pruritus, erythema, dryness and unbearable itching, infections and results with an impairment in quality of life [1-4]. For a long time, the mainstay of treatment for AD is the regular usage of emollient and topical anti-inflammatory medications (e.g., local or systemic steroids or other immunosuppressive agents) when needed [1, 2, 5, 6], which have been limited by their potential unwanted local or systemic side effects [7]. Complementary and alternative medicine (CAM) has gained popularity in the management of many chronic diseases, including AD [8]. Traditional Chinese medicine (TCM) is increasingly being used in the Western world, particularly in specialty areas such as gynecology, pediatrics, geriatrics, nutrition and dermatology. TCM is an alternative method of therapy that proposes to treat symptoms that Western medicine is unable to manage by reducing the underlying causes of disease and might cause less adverse effects [9]. One of the main drawbacks on the usage of TCM on AD treatment is that the beneficial effects on patients have not been consistently demonstrated, long-term effects of these agents are currently unavailable and undesirable side effects have been noted [10, 11].

Among some commonly used Chinese herbs in treating eczematous conditions with anti-allergic and anti-inflammatory activities and with no toxicity, we have chosen five herbs which was based on some widely used ancestral Chinese concoctions: Flos Lonicerae, Herba Menthae, Cortex Moutan, Rhizoma Atractylodis and Cortex Phellodendri to form an innovative PentaHerb Formula (PHF) for a systematic biological and clinical evaluation for AD treatment [12, 13].

CLINICAL TRIALS OF PHF

We have conducted a series of clinical studies to evaluate the efficacy, tolerability and dosage forms of PHF (Table 1). In a small scale pilot clinical test with nine children with AD for 28 days, we have evaluated the effects of PHF capsule [11].

Table 1. Clinical Trials of PentaHerbs Formula (PHF)

Clinical Trial	**Number of Patients**	**Outcomes/ References**
Open-labeled case series (2004) To evaluated the clinical and biochemical effects of a TCM capsule (PentaHerbs capsule) in children with AD.	9	No clinical or biochemical evidence of any adverse drug reaction was observed during the study period. The PentaHerbs capsules were well tolerated by the children and apparent beneficial effects were noted clinically. A larger, randomized placebo-controlled study is required to confirm the efficacy of this formulation for AD [11].
Randomized, double-blind, placebo-controlled study (2006) To assess the efficacy and tolerability of the concoction in children with AD.	85	The TCHM concoction is efficacious in improving quality of life and reducing topical corticosteroid use in children with moderate-to-severe AD. The formulation was palatable and well tolerated [15].
Open-label clinical trial (2007) To investigate the immunomodulatory effects that may be induced by PHF treatment.	28	Mean plasma concentrations of BDNF and TARC decreased significantly from 1798 pg/mL and 824 pg/mL at baseline to 1378 pg/mL and 492 pg/mL (P = 0.002 and 0.013, respectively) upon study completion. PHF possesses *in vitro* and *in vivo* immunomodulatory properties that may mediate the clinical efficacy observed in AD treatment [13].
Prospective self-controlled trial (2012) To evaluate the clinical efficacy and tolerability of the same concoction in syrup form.	22	The PHF syrup was generally palatable and well tolerated by the children. Adverse effects were generally mild but two patients with rash withdrew during the study. The palatability means that further evaluations and dosage studies of the concoction will be possible in young children [18, 21].

The capsules were manufactured, package by the Chinese Medicine Industry Development Centre, the Hong Kong Institute of Vocation Education, using the Good Manufacturing Practice (GMP) standard and hydrocortisone, prednisolone, fludrocortisone and dexamethasone were not detected in the PHF capsules [12]. Each capsule comprised 2 grams of Flos lonicerae, Cortex phellodendri, Cortex moutan, Rhizoma atractylodis and 1 gram of Herba menthae. Three PentaHerbs capsules twice a day were prescribed for four months with monthly follow up to ensure compliance, and SCORing Atopic Dermatitis (SCORAD) scores [14] were obtained at each visit. It was found that the PHF capsules were well tolerated by the children, there was significant improvement in the overall and component SCORAD scores from 60.3 to 40.0 for the patients and no adverse drug reaction was found [11].

To confirm the efficacy and tolerability of PHF, we have further conducted a larger placebo study [15]. 85 children with moderate-to-severe AD were randomized to receive a 12-week treatment with a twice-daily dose of 2 capsules of either PHF or placebo. The SCORAD score, Children's Dermatology Life Quality Index (CDLQI) [16], allergic rhinitis score, and the requirement for topical corticosteroid and oral antihistamine were assessed before and at weeks 4, 8, 12 and 16 of treatments. Adverse events, tolerability, hematological and biochemical parameters were monitored during the study. PHF was generally well tolerated and no significant difference in the frequency of adverse events reported by participants. Biochemical analysis also revealed no significant change in the IgE levels, complete blood counts, eosinophil counts, electrolytes, renal and liver functions. PHF was found to be efficacious in improving quality of life and reducing topical corticosteroids use in children with moderate-to-severe AD. The steroid sparing actions of PHF seems to be multi-targeted. PHF treatment resulted in a 15% reduction in the disease severity of the patients. Similar improvement was also noted in the placebo group during the study period but at the expense of more corticosteroid usage. We believed that the PHF might possess steroid-sparing and anti-inflammatory effects [17].

Inflammation plays an important role in AD pathogenesis, we further hypothesized that PHF possesses immunomodulatory activities that would account for its clinical efficacy in treating AD and we have another open-label clinical trial with 28 patients to evaluate the immunomodulatory effects of PHF in children with AD [13]. For the participants of the clinical trial, systemic corticosteroid, immunomodulating drug or TCM were stopped for at least 4 weeks before and throughout this clinical trial, and topical CS usage remained unchanged during the study. Three PHF capsules twice daily were prescribed for 3 months. Apart from full blood counts and biochemical safety tests (electrolytes, urea, creatinine, liver enzymes, bilirubin, bone profile and thyroid-stimulating hormone), two plasma inflammatory mediators implicated in AD immunopathology brain-derived neurotrophic factor (BDNF) and thymus- and activation-regulated chemokine (TARC) were measured. After 3 months, none of the patients had clinical or laboratory evidence of adverse events, the mean plasma concentrations of BDNF and TARC from the patients were decreased significantly from 1798 pg/mL and 824 pg/mL to 1378 pg/mL and 492 pg/mL, respectively [13]. These findings provide useful information to support the clinical benefits of PHF in treating AD.

AD is common in children who have difficulty swallowing whole capsules [18]. Therefore, PHF in capsule form may not be an ideal formulation for children. To cope with this situation, we have prepared PHF concoction in syrup for another prospective self-controlled trial [18]. Twenty-two children aged 4–7 years with moderate-to-severe AD received 20 ml of TCM syrup daily. After a 4-week treatment, there were significant improvements in the objective SCORAD, pruritus and CDLQI scores, no significant change in sleep score or amount of topical steroid consumption and no biochemical evidence of any adverse drug reaction was observed during the study period. The TCM syrup was generally palatable and well tolerated by the children, thereby suggesting that PHF in syrup form is suitable for children with beneficial effect in AD treatment. Apart from capsule and syrup formulation, direct topical formulation and herbal bath for PHF or other agents may also be useful in AD treatment, some pilot investigations are in progress [19, 20].

Laboratory Studies of PHF

Peripheral Blood Mononuclear Cells

The pathogenesis of AD involves complicated interactions among the host's environment such as skin barrier defects and immunological factors and immune cells, pharmacological abnormalities and susceptibility genes [13, 22]. A panel of inflammatory mediators were implicated in AD immunopathology, BDNF, TARC, interferon-gamma (IFN-γ) and tumor necrosis factor alpha (TNF-α) are some of the AD associated inflammatory cytokines. The beneficial effects of PHF in AD may be associated to immunomodulatory activities of PHF on different immune cells. Our laboratory studies showed that PHF could dose dependently suppress the proliferation of phytohaemagglutinin and Staphylococcal enterotoxin B (SEB)-stimulated peripheral blood mononuclear cells (PBMC) and productions of BDNF, TARC, IFN-γ and TNF-α, which was well correlated with our clinical study [13].

Mast Cells

Mast cells are known for their critical roles in AD attributed to their potent capability to produce multiple pro-inflammatory mediators including histamine, prostaglandins and cytokines after activation in allergic inflammation [23]. These mediators released from mast cells cause skin vasodilation, T-cell recruitment, inflammation and itching [1]. Inhibition of mast cells activation is a potential therapeutic strategy in AD. Using rat peritoneal mast cells, we found that PHF could potently inhibit histamine and prostaglandin D_2 release from both immunological activated mast cells, suggesting the clinical effect of PHF is related to the inhibition of mast cell activation [24]. Inhibitory actions of PHF on histamine and inflammatory cytokines such as TNF-α and CXCL8 from immunologically activated rat mast cells (MC) were also observed and the suppressive effect was mainly contributed by Cortex Moutan [24]. Cortex Moutan is known to have anti-allergic and anti-inflammatory properties and has been widely used in Asia for the treatment of atherosclerosis, infection, inflammation and cutaneous disease [25].

Dendritic Cells

Besides PBMC and mast cells, antigen-presentation to T cells is associated to allergic-inflammatory reactions in the pathogenesis of AD and it is performed by different antigen presenting dendritic cells (DC) subtypes bearing the high affinity receptor for IgE, such as Langerhans' cells and inflammatory dendritic epidermal cells [7]. Altered functions of DC in atopic individuals have been observed, especially the IDEC which have been suspected to play a major role in the generation and maintenance of inflammation by their production of large amounts of pro-inflammatory cytokines [26]. Monocytes are one of the precursors of DC and recent studies showed that monocytes rapidly infiltrate to inflamed tissues and mediates DC differentiation and contribute to the pathogenesis of AD [27, 28]. To stop the development of DC maturation from monocytes may offer a novel approach in the treatment of AD. We have fractionated the water crude extract of Cortex Moutan by high-speed counter-current chromatography (HSCCC) into 30 sub-fractions and we found that fraction 5 (F5) could dose dependently (50-200 μg/ml) inhibit IL-12-p40 and IL-10 from lipopolysaccharide (LPS)-activated monocyte-derived dendritic cells (moDC). Three active ingredients gallic acid, paeoniflorin and paeonol from Cortex Moutan were identified with immunosuppressive activities on immune cells [29-31]. DCs are specializing in the uptake, processing, transport and presentation of antigens to effector cells participating in both innate and adaptive immune systems. We have identified gallic acid as the major active ingredients from Cortex Moutan which could dose dependently inhibit IL-12-p40 and the functional surface marker expression such as CD40, CD80, CD83 and CD86 from cytokine cocktail-activated moDC [32]. We also found that gallic acid could lower the concentration of hydrocortisone required to inhibit the activation of DC. The results obtained in the DC study also in concordance with our clinical findings that PHF is efficacious in improving quality of life by reducing topical corticosteroids use in children with moderate-to-severe AD [15] .

Eosinophils

Infiltration of eosinophils into the dermal layer and presence of edema are typical characteristics in the skin biopsy of AD patients [33]. We have established two *in vitro* co-culture models which mimic the AD pathogenic environment: eosinophils and fibroblasts, and eosinophils and keratinocytes co-culture models which are useful for the pharmacological studies of anti-allergic compounds [34, 35]. Dermal fibroblast has been shown to induce maturation and promote the migration of DC. Allergen-specific IgG has also been shown to enhance secondary responses by ligating FcγRIII on DC and other antigen presenting cells to augment the development of Th2-mediated responses via an IL-33–dependent mechanism. Inhibition of this signaling pathway include AD-related cytokines/chemokines, cell surface expression of adhesion molecules and toll-like receptors, intercellular interaction and eosinophilic degranulation; the phosphorylation and activation of JAK-STAT, PI3K-AKT, MAPK and NF-κB pathways of DC/eosinophils and dermal fibroblasts may offer a novel approach of Th2-predominated AD.

We further found that two active ingredients of PHF: gallic acid and chlorogenic acid could suppress the release of AD-related pro-inflammatory cytokine IL-6 and chemokines CCL7 and CXCL8, respectively, in IL-31- and IL-33-treated eosinophils-dermal fibroblasts co-culture; another active ingredient berberine could suppress the release of AD-related IL-6, CXCL8, CCL2 and CCL7 in the eosinophil culture and eosinophils-dermal fibroblasts co-culture [36]. Murine study showed that ear swelling, epidermis thickening and eosinophils infiltration in epidermal and dermal layers, and the release of serum pro-inflammatory cytokines/chemokines of the murine oxazolone (OXA)-mediated dermatitis were significantly reduced upon oral or topical treatment with PHF. These findings suggest that PHF can ameliorate allergic inflammation and attenuate the activation of eosinophils [36].

Alteration of Gut Microbiome and Anti-Bacterial Activities of PHF

Regulatory T (Treg) cells are vital in the control of allergic responses in AD and asthma via immune suppression [37]. Gut microbiome has been found to play an important immunological role in modulating the activation of regulatory T cells (Treg) and the deactivation of dendritic cells in asthma murine model [38]. We have recently demonstrated that PHF could modulate the gut microbiome and the percentage of CD4+CD25highFoxp3+ Tregs in spleen [39]. Microbial DNA was extracted from the stool samples of the ovalbumin (OVA)-induced allergic asthmatic mice, and the hypervariable regions (V3-V4) of the 16S rRNA gene was sequenced using high-throughput Illumina HiSeq 2500. After the oral administration of PHF, the operational taxonomic units (OUTs) in the gut were increased by 1.22-fold in allergic asthmatic mice [39]. Changes in the gut microbiome composition were also observed at various taxonomic levels. While significantly reducing the abundance of the phylum Firmicutes; the 14-day PHF treatment significantly increases the abundance of putative asthma-protective Bacteroidetes in mice (all $p < 0.01$). Notably, the numbers of Lachnospiraceae bacterium 3-2 and Clostridium leptum were significantly reduced (all $p < 0.05$). On the other hand, the number of Clostridium sp. Culture-41 was remarkably increased upon a 14-day PHF treatment ($p < 0.01$). Moreover, PHF significantly elevated the abundance of Rhodospirillales, an order that comprises the acetic-acid-producing Acetobacteraceae family. These findings suggest that PHF can modulate the species composition and community structure of the gut microbiome in the OVA-induced allergic asthmatic mice. This study also reveals that alteration in gut microbiome may potentially contribute to the immunomodulatory activities of PHF in allergic diseases [39].

Innate immune defects in skin of patients suffered from AD make them more susceptible to secondary bacterial infection, especially *Staphylococcus aureus* colonization/infection [40] and the bacterial toxins serve as super antigens to augment cutaneous inflammation [41]. Gallic acid has been shown to inhibit the growth of *Staphylococcus aureus* and also drug resistant methicillin-resistant *Staphylococcus aureus* (MRSA) [42]. We found that PHF was effective against two tested strains: *Staphylococcus aureus* ATCC 25923 and MRSA ATCC BAA-43 and we suggested that PHF may be developed into a *Staphylococcus aureus* targeting topical application [43].

Development of PHF on Topical Therapy

The treatment of atopic dermatitis (AD) has long been viewed as a problematic issue by the medical profession. Although a wide variety of complementary therapies have been introduced, they fail to combine the skin moisturizing and drug supply for AD patients. Microencapsulation is defined as a technology for packaging materials in various forms in miniature, sealed capsules that can release their contents at controlled rates under specific conditions with an effective and long lasting method for the release of encapsulated drugs [44, 45]. Microencapsulation of PHF and/or its components and coated them to the garments for controlled releases of drugs to the skin could be good way for therapeutics application in AD treatment. By chitosan–sodium alginate (CSA) blend matrix and emulsion-chemical cross-linking method, we have successfully produced microcapsules loaded with PHF and Cortex Moutan (one of the component herb of PHF) respectively [20, 46, 47]. The microcapsules were of regular surface morphology, uniform particle size and displayed good controlled release of the herbal components over a long period of time. Cytotoxicity test showed that the CSA microcapsules do not have toxic effect on cells. CSA Herbal loaded microcapsule was successfully grafted onto the cotton fabrics.

We have also investigated other ways to coat PHF to garments. Mordant dyeing refers to the treatment of textile fabric with metallic salts or other complex forming agents which bind the natural mordantable dyes onto the textile [48]. By using different fibers mordant, PHF can be directly coated onto the fabrics [48]. Apart from drug direct delivery onto the skin, skin moisturizing is also important to relieve the symptoms of AD patients. To achieve this mission, we have successfully developed a fabricated P407/CMCs composite hydrogel system for both PHF/ Cortex Moutan delivery and moisturizing [49]. Hydrogel offers an ideal solution for developing this preconceived transdermal drug delivery system with dual-functions by its hydrophilic three-dimensional polymeric networks capable of absorbing a large amount of water or biological fluids [50]. Gallic acid, the active ingredient of Cortex Moutan, has been successfully incorporated into the drug delivery system of dual-responsive PF127 hydrogel with polysaccharide-based nano-conjugate for textile-based transdermal therapy with temperature and pH responsiveness for drug release [51].

CONCLUSION

Taking AD treatment as an example, we have attempted to adopt the historic and yet unique complementary medicine to become a safer and scientific-based therapy for wider applications.

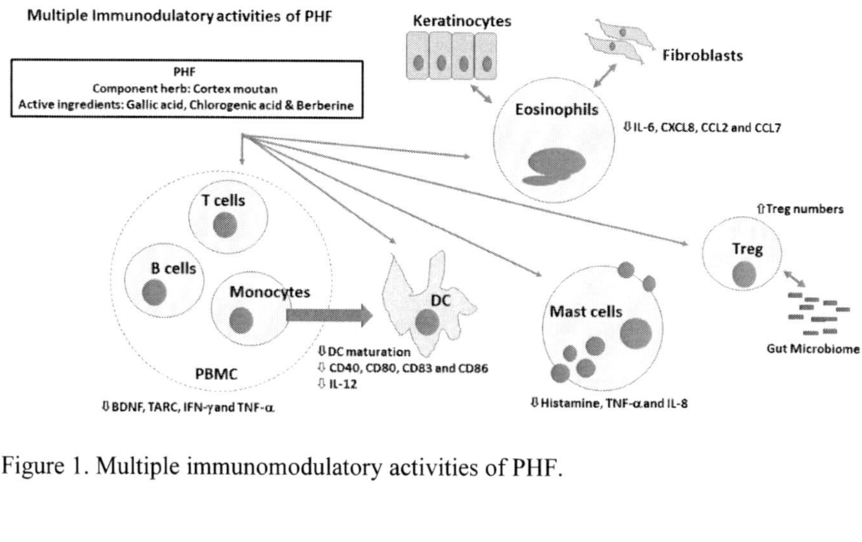

Figure 1. Multiple immunomodulatory activities of PHF.

From oral to topical, after a series of evidence-based clinical trials in compliance of Good Clinical Practice, we concluded that the PHF decoction is efficacious in improving quality of life and reducing topical corticosteroid use in children with moderate-to-severe AD. Both laboratory and clinical studies showed that the anti-inflammatory actions of PHF are multi-targeted (Figure 1) [13, 24, 32, 34, 36, 39, 43, 52]. We have also identified some active ingredients, namely, berberine, chlorogenic acid and gallic acid from PHF.

REFERENCES

[1] Leung AK, Hon KL, Robson WL: Atopic dermatitis. *Adv Pediatr* 2007, 54:241-273.

[2] Leung TN, Hon KL: Eczema therapeutics in children: what do the clinical trials say? *Hong Kong Med J* 2015, 21(3):251-260.

[3] Hon KL, Loo S, Leung AKC, Li JTS, Lee VWY: An overview of drug discovery efforts for eczema: why is this itch so difficult to scratch? *Expert Opin Drug Discov* 2020, 15(4):487-498.

[4] Hon KL, Chan BC, Leung PC: Chinese herbal medicine research in eczema treatment. *Chin Med* 2011, 6:17.

[5] van Zuuren EJ, Fedorowicz Z, Christensen R, Lavrijsen A, Arents BWM: Emollients and moisturisers for eczema. *Cochrane Database Syst Rev* 2017, 2:CD012119.

[6] Hon KL, Kung JSC, Ng WGG, Leung TF: Emollient treatment of atopic dermatitis: latest evidence and clinical considerations. *Drugs Context* 2018, 7:212530.

[7] Novak N, Kwiek B, Bieber T: The mode of topical immunomodulators in the immunological network of atopic dermatitis. *Clin Exp Dermatol* 2005, 30(2):160-164.

[8] Hon KL, Leung AKC, Leung TNH, Lee VWY: Complementary, Alternative and Integrative Medicine for Childhood Atopic Dermatitis. *Recent Pat Inflamm Allergy Drug Discov* 2017, 11(2):114-124.

[9] Baroni A, Ruocco E, Russo T, Piccolo V, Geng L, Zhou H, Chen HD, Gao XH: The use of traditional Chinese medicine in some dermatologic diseases: Part I--Acne, psoriasis, and atopic dermatitis. *Skinmed* 2015, 13(1):32-38; quiz 39.

[10] Hon KL, Leung AKC, Leung TNH, Lee VWY: Investigational drugs for atopic dermatitis. *Expert Opin Investig Drugs* 2018, 27(8):637-647.

[11] Hon KL, Leung TF, Wong Y, Lam WK, Guan DQ, Ma KC, Sung YT, Fok TF, Leung PC: A pentaherbs capsule as a treatment option for atopic dermatitis in children: an open-labeled case series. *Am J Chin Med* 2004, 32(6):941-950.

[12] Hon KL, Lee VW, Leung TF, Lee KK, Chan AK, Fok TF, Leung PC: Corticosteroids are not present in a traditional Chinese medicine formulation for atopic dermatitis in children. *Ann Acad Med Singapore* 2006, 35(11):759-763.

[13] Leung TF, Wong KY, Wong CK, Fung KP, Lam CW, Fok TF, Leung PC, Hon KL: In vitro and clinical immunomodulatory effects of a novel Pentaherbs concoction for atopic dermatitis. *Br J Dermatol* 2008, 158:1216-1223.

[14] Severity scoring of atopic dermatitis: the SCORAD index. Consensus Report of the European Task Force on Atopic Dermatitis. *Dermatology* 1993, 186(1):23-31.

[15] Hon KL, Leung TF, Ng PC, Lam MC, Kam WY, Wong KY, Lee KC, Sung YT, Cheng KF, Fok TF et al. Efficacy and tolerability of a Chinese herbal medicine concoction for treatment of atopic dermatitis: a randomized, double-blind, placebo-controlled study. *Br J Dermatol* 2007, 157(2):357-363.

[16] Lewis-Jones MS, Finlay AY: The Children's Dermatology Life Quality Index (CDLQI): initial validation and practical use. *Br J Dermatol* 1995, 132(6):942-949.

[17] Chen HY, Lin YH, Wu JC, Hu S, Yang SH, Chen JL, Chen YC, Lo SS: Use of traditional Chinese medicine reduces exposure to corticosteroid among atopic dermatitis children: a 1-year follow-up cohort study. *J Ethnopharmacol* 2015, 159:189-196.

[18] Hon KL, Lo W, Cheng WK, Leung TF, Chow CM, Lau CB, Fok TF, Ng PC, Leung PC: Prospective self-controlled trial of the efficacy and tolerability of a herbal syrup for young children with eczema. *J Dermatolog Treat* 2012, 23(2):116-121.

[19] Hon KL, Ng WGG, Kung JSC, Leung PC, Leung TF: Pilot Studies on Two Complementary Bath Products for Atopic Dermatitis Children: Pine-Tar and Tea. *Medicines (Basel)* 2019, 6(1).

[20] Hui PC, Wang WY, Kan CW, Ng FS, Wat E, Zhang VX, Chan CL, Lau CB, Leung PC: Microencapsulation of Traditional Chinese Herbs-PentaHerbs extracts and potential application in healthcare textiles. *Colloids Surf B Biointerfaces* 2013, 111:156-161.

[21] Hon KL, Lo W, Cheng WK, Leung TF, Chow CM, Lau CB, Fok TF, Ng PC, Leung PC: Prospective self-controlled trial of the efficacy and tolerability of a herbal syrup for young children with eczema. *J Dermatolog Treat* 2011, [Epub ahead of print].

[22] Leung DY: Atopic dermatitis: new insights and opportunities for therapeutic intervention. *J Allergy Clin Immunol* 2000, 105(5):860-876.

[23] Wang XS, Wu AY, Leung PS, Lau HY: PGE suppresses excessive anti-IgE induced cysteinyl leucotrienes production in mast cells of patients with aspirin exacerbated respiratory disease. *Allergy* 2007, 62(6):620-627.

[24] Chan BC, Hon KL, Leung PC, Sam SW, Fung KP, Lee MY, Lau HY: Traditional Chinese medicine for atopic eczema: PentaHerbs formula suppresses inflammatory mediators release from mast cells. *J Ethnopharmacol* 2008, 120(1):85-91.

[25] Hong MH, Kim JH, Na SH, Bae H, Shin YC, Kim SH, Ko SG: Inhibitory effects of Paeonia suffruticosa on allergic reactions by inhibiting the NF-kappaB/I kappaB-alpha signaling pathway and phosphorylation of ERK in an animal model and human mast cells. *Biosci Biotechnol Biochem* 2010, 74(6):1152-1156.

[26] Bieber T, Novak N, Herrman N, Koch S: Role of dendritic cells in atopic dermatitis: an update. *Clin Rev Allergy Immunol* 2011, 41(3):254-258.

[27] Leon B, Lopez-Bravo M, Ardavin C: Monocyte-derived dendritic cells formed at the infection site control the induction of protective T helper 1 responses against Leishmania. *Immunity* 2007, 26(4):519-531.

[28] Alonso MN, Wong MT, Zhang AL, Winer D, Suhoski MM, Tolentino LL, Gaitan J, Davidson MG, Kung TH, Galel DM et al. TH1, TH2, and TH17 cells instruct monocytes to differentiate into specialized dendritic cell subsets. *Blood* 2011, 118(12):3311-3320.

[29] Kim SH, Kim SA, Park MK, Kim SH, Park YD, Na HJ, Kim HM, Shin MK, Ahn KS: Paeonol inhibits anaphylactic reaction by regulating histamine and TNF-alpha. *Int Immunopharmacol* 2004, 4(2):279-287.

[30] Lee B, Shin YW, Bae EA, Han SJ, Kim JS, Kang SS, Kim DH: Antiallergic effect of the root of Paeonia lactiflora and its constituents paeoniflorin and paeonol. *Arch Pharm Res* 2008, 31(4):445-450.

[31] Kim SH, Jun CD, Suk K, Choi BJ, Lim H, Park S, Lee SH, Shin HY, Kim DK, Shin TY: Gallic acid inhibits histamine release and pro-inflammatory cytokine production in mast cells. *Toxicol Sci* 2006, 91(1):123-131.

[32] Chan BC, Li LF, Hu SQ, Wat E, Wong EC, Zhang VX, Lau CB, Wong CK, Hon KL, Hui PC et al. Gallic Acid Is the Major Active Component of Cortex Moutan in Inhibiting Immune Maturation of Human Monocyte-Derived Dendritic Cells. *Molecules* 2015, 20(9):16388-16403.

[33] Wong CK, Cheung PF, Ip WK, Lam CW: Interleukin-25-induced chemokines and interleukin-6 release from eosinophils is mediated by p38 mitogen-activated protein kinase, c-Jun N-terminal kinase, and nuclear factor-kappaB. *Am J Respir Cell Mol Biol* 2005, 33(2):186-194.

[34] Wong CK, Leung KM, Qiu HN, Chow JY, Choi AO, Lam CW: Activation of eosinophils interacting with dermal fibroblasts by pruritogenic cytokine IL-31 and alarmin IL-33: implications in atopic dermatitis. *PLoS One* 2012, 7(1):e29815.

[35] Cheung PF, Wong CK, Ho AW, Hu S, Chen DP, Lam CW: Activation of human eosinophils and epidermal keratinocytes by Th2 cytokine IL-31: implication for the immunopathogenesis of atopic dermatitis. *Int Immunol* 2010, 22(6):453-467.

[36] Tsang MS, Jiao D, Chan BC, Hon KL, Leung PC, Lau CB, Wong EC, Cheng L, Chan CK, Lam CW et al. Anti-Inflammatory Activities of Pentaherbs Formula, Berberine, Gallic Acid and Chlorogenic Acid in Atopic Dermatitis-Like Skin Inflammation. *Molecules* 2016, 21(4):519.

[37] Agrawal R, Wisniewski JA, Woodfolk JA: The role of regulatory T cells in atopic dermatitis. *Curr Probl Dermatol* 2011, 41:112-124.

[38] Kamada N, Nunez G: Role of the gut microbiota in the development and function of lymphoid cells. *J Immunol* 2013, 190(4):1389-1395.

[39] Tsang MS, Cheng SW, Zhu J, Atli K, Chan BC, Liu D, Chan HY, Sun X, Chu IM, Hon KL et al. Anti-Inflammatory Activities of Pentaherbs formula and Its Influence on Gut Microbiota in Allergic Asthma. *Molecules* 2018, 23(11).

[40] Hon KL, Wang SS, Lee KK, Lee VW, Leung TF, Ip M: Combined antibiotic/corticosteroid cream in the empirical treatment of moderate to severe eczema: friend or foe? *J Drugs Dermatol* 2012, 11(7):861-864.

[41] Homey B, Steinhoff M, Ruzicka T, Leung DY: Cytokines and chemokines orchestrate atopic skin inflammation. *J Allergy Clin Immunol* 2006, 118(1):178-189.

[42] Shibata H, Nakano T, Parvez MA, Furukawa Y, Tomoishi A, Niimi S, Arakaki N, Higuti T: Triple combinations of lower and longer alkyl gallates and oxacillin improve antibiotic synergy against methicillin-resistant *Staphylococcus aureus*. *Antimicrobial agents and chemotherapy* 2009, 53(5):2218-2220.

[43] Hon KL, Ip M, Wong CK, Chan BCL, Leung PC, Leung TF: In vitro antimicrobial effects of a novel Pentaherbs concoction for atopic dermatitis. *J Dermatolog Treat* 2018, 29(3):235-237.

[44] Opara EC: Applications of Cell Microencapsulation. *Methods Mol Biol* 2017, 1479:23-39.

[45] Nelson G: Application of microencapsulation in textiles. *Int J Pharm* 2002, 242(1-2):55-62.

[46] Patrick CLH, Frency SFN, CWK, Wenyi W, Change Z, PCL, Clara B-SL, Elaine W, Ben CLC: Empirical Study of developing microcapsules with herbal extract for clinical treatment. *Journal of Textile Engineering* 2013, 59(5):99-103.

[47] Hui PC, Wang WY, Kan CW, Zhou CE, Ng FS, Wat E, Zhang VX, Chan CL, Lau CB, Leung PC: Preparation and characterisation of chitosan microcapsules loaded with Cortex Moutan. *Int J Biol Macromol* 2013, 55:32-38.

[48] Wang W, Wat E, Hui PCL, Ng FSF, Kan CW, Wong ECW, Chan B, Lau CBS, Leung P-C: Application of Chinese herbal medicine onto cotton fabric by dyeing methods. *Fibers and Polymers* 2015, 16(11):2401-2408.

[49] Wang W, Hui PCL, Wat E, Ng FSF, Kan CW, Wang X, Wong ECW, Hu H, Chan B, Lau CBS et al. In vitro drug release and percutaneous behavior of poloxamer-based hydrogel formulation containing traditional Chinese medicine. *Colloids Surf B Biointerfaces* 2016, 148:526-532.

[50] Lin CC, Metters AT: Hydrogels in controlled release formulations: network design and mathematical modeling. *Adv Drug Deliv Rev* 2006, 58(12-13):1379-1408.

[51] Chatterjee S, Hui PC, Wat E, Kan CW, Leung PC, Wang W: Drug delivery system of dual-responsive PF127 hydrogel with polysaccharide-based nano-conjugate for textile-based transdermal therapy. *Carbohydr Polym* 2020, 236:116074.

[52] Liu KY, Hu S, Chan BC, Wat EC, Lau CB, Hon KL, Fung KP, Leung PC, Hui PC, Lam CW et al. Anti-inflammatory and anti-allergic activities of Pentaherb formula, Moutan Cortex (Danpi) and gallic acid. *Molecules* 2013, 18(3):2483-2500.

In: Atopic Dermatitis
Editor: Andreas Maur
ISBN: 978-1-53618-520-1

Chapter 7

THE USE OF TOPICAL CORTICOSTEROIDS IN MANAGEMENT OF ATOPIC DERMATITIS AND THE ADVERSE EFFECTS

Yik-Ling Chew, Mayasah Al-Nema and Vivian Wai-Mun Ong
Department of Pharmaceutical Chemistry,
UCSI University, Kuala Lumpur

ABSTRACT

Atopic dermatitis (AD) also known as atopic eczema or eczema. It is a chronic inflammatory, pruritic skin disease that significantly affected the quality of life (QOL) for both patients and families. Topical corticosteroids (TCS) are commonly used by dermatologists and general physicians to treat selected difficult dermatoses effectively. The available range of formulations and potency gives flexibility to treat all groups of patients, different phases of disease, and different anatomic sites. However, majority people are afraid when come to TCS treatments. This fear is due to side effects of improper use of TCS by dermatologists, general physicians, and patients. To maximise therapeutic benefit and minimize the adverse effect, it is necessary to consider the choice of TCS during the diagnosis as well as steroid potency, delivery vehicle, frequency of administration, duration of treatment, and side effects. Benefits of rational and ethical use, danger of overuse and misuse for non-medical, especially for cosmetic purposes, should be clearly evaluate before prescription.

INTRODUCTION

Atopic dermatitis (AD) is an inflammatory skin illness that characterize by pruritic, erythematous, scaly papules, vesicles, and plaques that might continue as chronic lichenified lesions caused by water loss through the epidermis, intense itching, and cutaneous inflammation.[1, 2]. The term AD is frequently used interchangeably with eczema.

Atopic means, tendency to have elevated serum of immunoglobulin E (IgE) antibodies. AD usually affect 60 – 80% of patients and a personal or family history of type 1 allergies, allergic rhinitis, and asthma [3, 4]. AD is categorized into two types, asymptomatic sensitization (outside-to-inside) and non-sensitized (inside-to-outside). In asymptomatic sensitization, it is due to defect in skin barrier where the allergens can easily enter into the epidermal and cause secondary immunologic reaction, it is usually triggered by the environment such as pollen, house dust mite, and food allergens [5]. As for non-sensitized it is normally concomitant with allergy, asthma and stress [6].

The physical effect usually affects the routine activities of the patients (e.g., school, work, sleep), and patients can experience distress and worry, that weakens their psychological wellbeing and functional capacity. Management for AD is effective at easing the symptoms and is vital to avoid complications, such as infection, sleep disturbance, behavioural problems, and psychosocial strain.

There are a few methods in management of AD, such as daily intervention, emollients and topical therapy [5]. Daily intervention and emollients are usually use for the prevention of the reoccurring of AD while topical therapy are more towards the medical treatment for diagnosis [5, 7].

To date, the most effective management therapy for AD conditions are topical corticosteroids (TCS) because they specifically target hyperproliferation, inflammation, and immunologic response [8]. TCS are introduced since 1952 by Sulzberger and Witten. It is the most important breakthrough in the history of therapy of dermatological disorders [9]. Even though TCS have greatly contributed to dermatologist's ability to treat several difficult dermatoses [10], there are still an argument pertaining the good and bad of TCS as effective management therapy due to the various harmful side effects. Research study showed that approximate 72.5% of TCS users were worried about the side effects, such as Cushing's syndrome, cutaneous and ocular side effects [11]. Cushing's syndrome due to the prolonged usage of high potency TCS could suppress the hypothalamopituitory-adrenal axis in children. Skin thinning (atrophy), stretch marks (striae), easy bruising and tearing of the skin, enlarged blood vessels (telangiectasia) and localised increased hair thickness and length (hypertrichosis) are the common cutaneous side effects. Excessive use of TCS on eyelid skin may result in ocular side effects including glaucoma or cataracts.

TOPICAL CORTICOSTEROIDS (TCS)

TCS is a synthetic cortisol drugs that resemble the natural cortisol produce in the body. They work by relieving inflammation and they have immunosuppressive properties [1]. They can also provide symptomatic relief for burning and pruritic lesions [8]. TCS can be lifesaving with many benefits. However, its therapeutic usage must be optimised to avoid any potential risks and serious adverse effects. Hence, the choice of TCS during the diagnosis, including the steroid potency, delivery vehicle, frequency of administration, duration of treatment, and potential side effects must be meticulously considered. This is to ensure that the therapeutic benefit of TCS selected for the treatment could be maximised, with minimum adverse effects [8, 12].

Potency of Topical Corticosteroids and Their Uses

The available range of formulations and potency gives flexibility to treat all groups of patients, different phases of disease, and different anatomic sites. There are many TCS available and they are classified according to potency (least, low, medium, high and ultra-high). Table 1 is the common type of TCS in their respective potency strength.

Table 1. Potency Ratings of Topical Corticosteroids

Potency	Topical corticosteroid
Least potent (VII)	Hydrocortisone 1%, 2.5%
Low (VI)	Alclometasone dipropionate 0.05%, Desonide 0.05%, Fluocinolone 0.01%, Hydrocortisone butyrate 0.1%
Medium (IV and V)	Betamethasone valerate, Desoximetasone 0.05%, Fluocinolone acetonide 0.025%, Fluticasone propionate 0.05%, Hydrocortisone butyrate 0.1%, Hydrocortisone probutate 0.1%, Hydrocortisone valerate 0.2%, Mometasone furoate 0.1%
Medium to high (III)	Amcinonide 0.1%, Betamethasone dipropionate 0.05%, Fluticasone propionate 0.005%, Triamcinolone acetonide 0.5%
High (II)	Amcinonide 0.1%, Augmented betamethasone dipropionate 0.05%, Betamethasone dipropionate 0.05%, Desoximetasone, Diflorasone diacetate 0.05%, Fluocinonide 0.05%
Ultra-high (I)	Augmented betamethasone dipropionate 0.05%, Clobetasol propionate 0.05%, Diflorasone diacetate 0.05%, Fluocinonide 0.1%, Flurandrenolide 4 mcg per m^2, Halobetasol propionate 0.05%

TCS of least to medium potency are particularly suitable for the treatment of AD in areas where the skin is sensitive and thin, such as the neck, genitals, the face, the back of the knees, the insides of the elbows, the groin area and the armpits. Medium-to high-potency TCS are effective for AD in adults and children [2, 13], as well as for phimosis (foreskin that cannot be retracted) [14] and acute radiation dermatitis [15]. High-potency and ultra-high-potency corticosteroids are used for the treatment of severe cases on the palms of the hands, soles of the feet, and areas with very thick skin. They should not be used on the face, groin, axilla, or under occlusion, except in rare situations and for short durations.

Delivery Vehicle of TCS

The vehicles for TCS available including cream, ointment, gel, lotion and solution [8].

Creams

Creams are the mixtures of oil and water. They have good lubricating qualities, and their ability to vanish into the skin makes them cosmetically appealing. Creams are generally less potent than ointments of the same medication, and they often contain preservatives, which can cause irritation, stinging, and allergic reaction. Creams are also useful in intertriginous areas where ointments may not be used. However, creams do not provide the occlusive effects that ointments provide.

Ointments

Ointments provide more lubrication and occlusion than other preparations. They are translucent and greasy, hence are the most useful for application to dry or thick, hyperkeratotic lesion. Their occlusive nature also improves steroid absorption. Ointments should not be used on hairy areas. They may cause maceration and folliculitis if used on intertriginous areas (e.g., groin, gluteal cleft, axilla).

Gels and Lotions

Gels and lotions are more suitable for exudative lesion, body areas which are protected by hair and less exposed. These areas are usually moister. Hydration generally promotes TCS penetration and absorption and therefore the potency is enhanced. These types of delivery vehicle are best for scalp and other hair covered areas. Their occlusive nature also improves absorption. Lotions and gels are the least greasy and occlusive of all topical steroid vehicles. Lotions are useful for hairy areas because they penetrate easily. Gels have a jelly-like consistency and are beneficial for exudative inflammation. Gels generally dry quickly and can be applied on the scalp or other hairy areas.

Frequency of Administration and Duration of Treatment

Once or twice-daily application is suggested for most preparations. During maintenance treatment, TCS can be applied to "hotspots" twice per week [16]. Frequent application may not necessary offer better results. The best dosing guidelines is by trial and error, titrating to the least frequency of application that provides relief [17].

Chronic application of TCS can bring tolerance and tachyphylaxis. Therefore, ultra-high-potency TCS must not apply for more than three weeks continuously. If a longer period is required, the TCS should be slowly tapered to prevent rebound symptoms. Then, treatment is continued after a steroid-free period, at least one week after. This alternating schedule can repeat regularly until the condition relief. Side effects are rare when low-to-high-potency TCS are used for three months or less, except in intertriginous and occlusion area, on the neck and face.

APPLICATION DOSAGE: ONE FINGERTIP UNIT (FTU) METHOD AND RULE OF HAND

A standardized 'fingertip unit (FTU)' and 'rule of hand' have been invented to measure the amount of ointment required to cover specific anatomic areas adequately [18, 19]. FTU is the amount of TCS ointment expressed from a nozzle with 5 mm diameter, applied from the distal skin crease to the top of the palmar aspect of the index finger [18]. The 'rule of hand' is the area of one side of a flat closed hand requires approximately 0.5 fingertip units, which is also equivalent to 0.25 g ointment [19]. Jonathan [17] had reported the fingertip unit required for one application as follows (1 FTU equivalent to 0.5 g, approximately).

- Face and neck: 2.5 FTU
- Trunk (front and back): 7 FTU
- One arm: 3 FTU
- One hand (one side): 0.5 FTU
- One leg: 6 FTU
- One foot: 2 FTU

ADVERSE EFFECTS OF TCS

Adverse effects occur more often with prolong use of higher potencies TCS [20]. To minimize the adverse effects, TCS with the least potency should be firstly used before higher potency TCS are considered. The duration of TCS usage should be as minimum as possible. This is to maintain its effectiveness and lower the adverse effects of TCS. The application of high potency TCS i.e., clobetasol and halobetasol propionate should not exceed 14 days [21]. The total dose of halobetasol should not be used more than 50 gm/week and clobetasol should not be use more than 60 gm/week. Table 2 summarized the local side effects of TCS with associated risk factors and mechanism.

Table 2. Lists the local side effects of TCS with associated risk factors and mechanism

Unwanted effects of topical steroids	Clinical features	Risk factors and mechanism
Epidermal effects	Epidermal thinning	Decrease in mean keratinocytes layer thickness Flattening of the dermo epidermal convolutions Decrease in epidermal kinetic activity
	Melanocyte inhibition (vitiligo like condition)	Intradermal steroid injections, steroids under occlusion
Dermal effects	Striae	Risk factors
	Easy rupture on trauma	Young age
	Blot haemorrhage	Potency of steroid
	Stellate scars	Use of occlusion
	Prematurely aged skin appearance	Location (face, neck, axilla, groin, upper inner thigh) Decrease in ground substance and collagen synthesis
Combined epidermal and dermal effects	Atrophy Telangiectasia Striae Purpura Stellate pseudoscars Ulceration Easy bruising	Dermal atrophy and loss of intercellular substance, causing blood vessels to lose their surrounding dermal matrix
Vascular effects	Fixed vasodilation Rebound phenomenon Perioral dermatitis Rosacea Facial erythema	

Unwanted effects of topical steroids	**Clinical features**	**Risk factors and mechanism**
Ocular effects	Due to steroid eye drops Glaucoma/cataract Decrease healing of traumatic ulcers Exacerbation of herpetic ulcer Increased susceptibility to bacterial and fungal infections Blindness (on prolonged use) Few side effects due to topical steroids applied around eyes Blindness due to glaucoma after long term steroid on face	
Contact allergy	Allergic or irritant contact dermatitis	Risk factors History of many positive patch test to nontopical steroid allergen Treatment resistant eczema Leg ulcers Stasis dermatitis Perineal dermatitis
Infections	Exacerbation on increased susceptibility to bacterial, viral and fungal infections (e.g., Candidiasis, herpes or Demodex) Folliculitis Crusted scabies Granuloma gluteal infantum, genital ulceration Masking of microbial infections (tinea incognito) and (tinea pseudoimbricata)	

Table 2. (Continued)

Unwanted effects of topical steroids	Clinical features	Risk factors and mechanism
Effect on hair	Hypertrichosis (prevalent on face and ears) Lanugo hair Alopecia	
Vehicle related effects	Stinging Irritation Folliculitis Miliaria Exacerbation of acne and rosacea Allergic contact dermatitis	
Pharmacologic effects	Tachyphylaxis	Risk factors Patient noncompliance Normal variance in disease severity that is unrelated to therapy Inability of steroids to completely clear the disease
	Steroid rebound Steroid addiction	

Unwanted effects of topical steroids	**Clinical features**	**Risk factors and mechanism**
Miscellaneous	Acneiform eruption	Comedone formation by rendering follicular epithelium more responsive to comedogenesis Increased concentration of free fatty acids in skin surface lipids and increased number of bacteria in the pilosebaceous duct
	Miliaria Urticaria Delayed wound healing Tachyphylaxis Reactivation of Kaposi's sarcoma Alternation of fat distribution (Cushingoid appearance) Hypopigmentation (common in dark skinned and reversible) Hyperpigmentation Rebound flare (psoriasis)	
	Milia	Risk factors Long term use Old age

Reproduced from Coondoo, et al. [22].

The most frequently reported adverse effects of TCS are local irritation (66%), skin discoloration (15%), and striae or skin atrophy (15%) [20]. Other effects were also reported, such as rosacea and other pharmacological effect including tachyphylaxis, rebound phenomenon, steroid addiction, wound healing inhibition and epidermal barrier disturbance [22].

Local Irritation

Local irritation such as burning or stinging of the skin is a common effect when treatment started. This skin irritation is could be due to worsening of a pre-existing skin infection and folliculitis, an inflamed hair follicles and thinning of skin that causes the skin more vulnerable to damage such as bruise [22]. There was study that indicate TCS may induce skin irritation, while others reported that the skin irritation could be due to the antiproliferative effect of TCS in delaying skin barrier regeneration [22].

Atrophy Changes

Atrophy of the epidermis and dermis is one of the common adverse effects of using TCS. Atrophic changes can affect both epidermis and dermis where stratum granulosum disappears and stratum corneum becomes thin. This is due to the reduction of epidermal cell size and reduction in metabolic activity. The skin of delicate sites such as the eyelids will be more likely to atrophy from even mild-potency TCS. The application of mild potency TCS to the eyelids could cause serious local adverse effect such as glaucoma [23-25]. In addition, the application of TCS on occlusion area, face, back of the hands and intertriginous area may also have higher risk of atrophy [17].

Various atrophy changes could be noticed as the effect of TCS usage, including telangiectasia, striae, hyperpigmentation and hypopigmentation (Table 3).

Table 3. Atrophy changes and the appearance of skin

Atrophy changes	Appearance of skin
Telangiectasia	Tiny blood vessels appear threadlike red lines on the skin.
Striae	Flattened, thinned skin with a pink hue that can be pruritic. It may enlarge in length and width, appeared reddish purple in colour. The surface of striae may be finely wrinkled.
Purpura and stellate pseudoscars	The blood vessels lose the surrounding dermal matrix resulting lesions damage such as purpuric, irregularly shaped, hypopigmented, depressed scars.
Hypopigmentation	Light skinned individuals are caused by the interference with the melanin synthesis by smaller melanocytes, causing patchy areas of hypopigmentation. Hypopigmentation is due to the inhibition of melanocytes functions.
Hyperpigmentation	Patches of skin become darker than normal surrounding skin. This darkening occurs when an excess of melanin synthesis.

ROSACEA

Prolonged use of TCS may cause rosacea on the face, especially in middle aged woman, where papules and pustules are seen in patients. TCS-induced rosacea is characterized by centrofacial, perioral, and periocular monomorphic inflammatory papules and pustules in areas that have been chronically exposed to TCS [26]. Other symptoms include burning and stinging sensations, permanent redness, spots (papules and pustules), visible of small blood vessels in the skin. Rosacea is a relapsing condition (rebound symptoms). The symptoms may possibly turn bad when it flare-up [27]. If the symptoms persist and TCS potency is progressively increased, rosacea may become refractory to further treatment and hence the use of TCS must be discontinued [26]. This may cause a severe rebound erythema and pustule out-break [8, 27].

Tachyphylaxis

Tachyphylaxis is the decreasing efficacy of TCS during continued treatment. This is due to the reduction in sensitivity of the tissues which will normally result in the usage of higher potency TCS [28]. Tachyphylaxis occurred to vasoconstrictive and DNA-suppressing effects of TCS [29]. This can be quantified by vasoconstrictor assay and inhibition of fibroblast proliferation [28].

Rebound Phenomenon

Studies had showed that rebound phenomenon after regression from TCS [30-33]. Withdrawal of potent TCS for a prolonged period may result in a relapse or a papulopustular flare and may cause unstable or severe generalized pustular psoriasis [28]. Kimata [34] studied the serum levels of cytokines during the rebound phenomenon. It was found that increase in cytokines such as IL-4, IL-5, IL-10 and IL-13. These cytokines are synthesized by Th2. No change in cytokines produced by Th1, such as IL-2 and IFN-γ.

Topical Corticosteroid Addiction

TCS addiction is also known as red burning skin syndrome [35]. TCS addiction is the situation in which the symptoms became worse than pre-treatment after withdrawal [36]. Clinical findings described that the addicted skin is well-controlled under TCS. However, itching may be more uncomfortable than before TCS treatment or some may find the efficiency of TCS reduced. Prurigo-like eruptions developed as intractable lesions after taking TCS in some patients. Dermatologists explained that prurigo as a chronic and difficult-to-treat type of eruption observed in patients could be the sign of TCS addiction [35]. Spreading of eruption to other areas of the skin where TCS are not previously applied, i.e., extending from face to the neck, from upper extremities to lower extremities, from finger to the arms [35].

Delay in Wound Healing

Wound healing is a complex biological process that involves inflammatory cells proliferation to the wound, granulation of tissue formation, epithelial closure, cell differentiation, matrix deposition and remodelling. The wound healing process involves variety of growth factors and cytokines [37, 38]. The frequent use of TCS on AD could delay the wound healing process. TCS consist of the main armamentarium that could control the symptoms of ulcerous and inflammation [39]. The long-term usage of TCS could suppress the wound healing process. The delay in wound healing process is caused by inhibition of keratinocytes, fibroblasts, vascular connective tissue and angiogenesis. Inhibition of keratinocytes would impair or delay the re-epithelialization process. Inhibition of fibroblasts resulted in reduction of collagen and ground substance may cause dermal atrophy and formation of striae [40]. Inhibition of vascular connective tissue will result in telangiectasia and purpura. The process of delayed granulation tissue and inhibition of angiogenesis are also the cause of delayed wound healing [40, 41].

Epidermal Barrier Disturbance

TCS exhibit inhibitory effects on lipid precursor synthesis in keratinocytes and impairments of the lamellar structure in the stratum corneum [42] which resulted in epidermal barrier disturbance. TCS have been reported could suppress the mitosis and DNA synthesis in keratinocytes, which resulted in thinning of the epidermis [43-45]. Besides inhibition of stratum corneum neutral lipids, suppression of involucrin and filaggrin are also noticed in atrophic skin [42, 45]. These processes could result in significant increase in transepidermal water loss (TEWL) due to the impairment of epidermal barrier [45]. The barrier disruption is also contributing directly to the rebound phenomenon.

Optimizing the Use of TCS

The usage of TCS including the frequency, strength and appropriateness should be carefully optimised. Suitable strength of TCS should be based on the conditions of the skin. The strength and frequency of the usage should be reduced when the skin conditions improved. In addition, precautions should always be taken when TCS is prescribed for certain body areas, such as face, flexures and genital areas

The usage, potency and dosage of TCS used should be carefully optimized based on the recommendation by dermatologists and doctors, as follows.

- suitable potency and strength to reach disease control
- maintain less potent prescription or reduce frequency of application when condition get better, extra precaution should be taken when prescribing TCS over certain locations (e.g., scrotum, face, and flexures) and to the elderly and children
- awareness on the adverse effects and act immediately to counteract them
- avoid homemade dilutions of TCS and prescribing TCS in combination with antimicrobial and antifungal
- resist temptation to use TCS for an undiagnosed rash.

Conclusion

TCS are still the most effective treatment in the management of AD [9, 46]. However, it is increasingly apparent that TCS are being misused by doctors and patients [17]. Extra precautions should be taken when they are prescribed and used. TCS are generally safe to be used if they are used appropriately and correctly.

REFERENCES

[1] Weissler, Anne. "Atopic Dermatitis–a New Dawn." *Physician Assistant Clinics* 1, no. 4 (2016): 661-82.

[2] Hanifin, J., A. K. Gupta, and R. Rajagopalan. "Intermittent Dosing of Fluticasone Propionate Cream for Reducing the Risk of Relapse in Atopic Dermatitis Patients." *Br J Dermatol* 147, no. 3 (2002): 528-37.

[3] Eichenfield, Lawrence F, Wynnis L, Tom, Sarah L, Chamlin "Guidelines of Care for the Management of Atopic Dermatitis." *J Am Acad Dermatol* 70, no. 2 (2014): 338-51.

[4] Reitamo S, Malcolm R, Thomas R, Frederic C, Kirsti K. "Efficacy and Safety of Tacrolimus Ointment Compared with That of Hydrocortisone Butyrate Ointment in Adult Patients with Atopic Dermatitis." *J Allergy Clinical Immunol* 109, no. 3 (2001): 547-55.

[5] Chew, Yik-Ling, Mayasah Al-Nema, and Vivian Wai-Mun Ong. "Management and Treatment of Atopic Dermatitis with Modern Therapies, Complementary and Alternative Medicines: A Review." *Oriental Pharmacy and Experimental Medicine* 18, no. 2 (2018): 67-76.

[6] KH, Kim. "Overview of Atopic Dermatitis." *Asia Pacific Allergy* 3, no. 2 (2013): 79-87.

[7] Judith H, Joerg B, Timothy GB and Martin S. "Management of Itch in Atopic Dermatitis." *Semin Cutan Med Surg* 30, no. 2 (2013): 71-86.

[8] D, Jonathan. "Choosing Topical Corticosteroids." *Am Fam Physician* 79, no. 2 (2009): 135-40.

[9] Sulzberger, MB., and VH. Witten. "The Effect of Topically Applied Compound F in Selected Dermatoses." *J Invest Dermatol* 19, no. 2 (1952): 101-2.

[10] D, Sanjay K. Rathi and Paschal. "Rational and Ethical Use of Topical Corticosteroids Based on Safety and Efficacy." *Indian J Dermatol* 57, no. 4 (2012): 251-59.

[11] Charman, CR, AD Morris, and Willimes HC. "Topical Corticosteroid Phobia in Patients with Atopic Eczema." *British Journal of Dermatology* 142 (1999): 931-36.

[12] Ffrooz A, Tehranchia-nia Z, Ahmed AR. "Benefits and Risks of Intralesional Corticosteroid Injection in the Treatment of Dermatological Diseases." *Clinical and experimental dermatology* 20 (1995): 363-70.

[13] Tan, MH., SL. Meador, G. Singer, and MG. Lebwohl. "An Open-Label Study of the Safety and Efficacy of Limited Application of Fluticasone Propionate Ointment, 0.005%, in Patients with Atopic Dermatitis of the Face and Intertriginous Areas." *Int J Dermatol* 41, no. 11 (2002): 804-9.

[14] Lund, L., KH. Wai, LM. Mui, and CK. Yeung. "Effect of Topical Steroid on Non-Retractile Prepubertal Foreskin by a Prospective, Randomized, Double-Blind Study." *Scandinavian Journal of Urology and Nephrology* 34, no. 4 (2000): 267-69.

[15] Schmuth, M., MA. Wimmer, S. Hofer, A. Sztankay, G. Weinlich, D. M. Linder, PM. Elias, PO. Fritsch, and E. Fritsch. "Topical Corticosteroid Therapy for Acute Radiation Dermatitis: A Prospective, Randomized, Double-Blind Study." *Br J Dermatol* 146, no. 6 (2002): 983-91.

[16] Diana, R, T Thiru, WS Retno, CKW Steven, MG Teresita, LV Lillian, C Chia-Yu, D Sandipan, P Deepak, W Li-Chuen, and L Kuen-Kong. *Journal of Dermatology. Consensus guidelines for the management of atopic dermatitis: An Asia–Pacific perspective* 40 (2013): 160-71.

[17] Jonathan, DF. "Choosing Topical Corticosteroids." *American Academy of Family Physicians* 79, no. 2 (2009): 135-40.

[18] Long, CC, and AY Finlay. "The Finger-Tip Unit—a New Practical Measure." *Clinical and experimental dermatology* 16, no. 6 (1991): 444-47.

[19] Long, CC, AY Finlay, and RW Averill. "The Rule of Hand: 4 Hand Areas= 2 Ftu= 1 G." *Archives of dermatology* 128, no. 8 (1992): 1129-30.

[20] Wahane, P, R Jagtap, and B Ghongane. "Evaluation of Corticosteroid Use Pattern in Steroid Responsive Dermatological Conditions." *Int J Med Res Health Sci* 5 (2016): 82-86.

[21] Mehta, Aayushi B, Nitin J Nadkarni, Sharmila P Patil, Kiran V Godse, Manjyot Gautam, and Shweta Agarwal. "Topical Corticosteroids in Dermatology." *Indian Journal of Dermatology, Venereology, and Leprology* 82, no. 4 (2016): 371.

[22] Coondoo, A., M. Phiske, S. Verma, and K. Lahiri. "Side-Effects of Topical Steroids: A Long Overdue Revisit." *Indian Dermatol Online J* 5, no. 4 (2014): 416-25.

[23] Cubey, R Bevis. "Glaucoma Following the Application of Corticosteroid to the Skin of the Eyelids." *British Journal of Dermatology* 95, no. 2 (1976): 207-08.

[24] Zugerman, Charles, Donald Sauders, and Fred Levit. "Glaucoma from Topically Applied Steroids." *Archives of dermatology* 112, no. 9 (1976): 1326-26.

[25] Nielsen, Niels V, and Per N Sørensen. "Glaucoma Induced by Application of Corticosteroids to the Periorbital Region." *Archives of dermatology* 114, no. 6 (1978): 953-54.

[26] Bhat, Yasmeen J, Sheikh Manzoor, and Seema Qayoom. "Steroid-Induced Rosacea: A Clinical Study of 200 Patients." *Indian journal of dermatology* 56, no. 1 (2011): 30.

[27] *Rosacea Is a Common but Poorly Understood Long-Term Skin Condition That Mainly Affects the Face.* http://www.nhs.uk/conditions/Rosacea/Pages/Introduction.aspx (accessed 16-November-2016).

[28] Coondoo A, Phiske M, Verma S, Lahiri K. "Side-Effects of Topical Steroids: A Long Overdue Revisit." *Indian Dermatology Online Journal.* 5, no. 4 (2014): 416-25.

[29] Czarnowicki, Tali, Rita V Linkner, Mayte Suárez-Fariñas, Arie Ingber, and Mark Lebwohl. "An Investigator-Initiated, Double-Blind,

Vehicle-Controlled Pilot Study: Assessment for Tachyphylaxis to Topically Occluded Halobetasol 0.05% Ointment in the Treatment of Psoriasis." *Journal of the American Academy of Dermatology* 71, no. 5 (2014): 954-59. e1.

[30] Forte, WC Neves, J Mayumi Sumita, A Gianini Rodrigues, D Liuson, and E Tanaka. "Rebound Phenomenon to Systemic Corticosteroid in Atopic Dermatitis." *Allergologia et immunopathologia* 33, no. 6 (2005): 307-11.

[31] Wells, Kenneth, and Robert T Brodell. "Topical Corticosteroid 'Addiction' a Cause of Perioral Dermatitis." *Postgraduate medicine* 93, no. 5 (1993): 225-30.

[32] Fukuyama, Tomoki, Joy Rachel Ganchingco, and Wolfgang Bäumer. "Demonstration of Rebound Phenomenon Following Abrupt Withdrawal of the Jak1 Inhibitor Oclacitinib." *European journal of pharmacology* 794 (2017): 20-26.

[33] Sarkar, Rashmi, and Nisha V Parmar. "Topical Side Effects of Topical Corticosteroids." In *A Treatise on Topical Corticosteroids in Dermatology*, 251-60: Springer, 2018.

[34] Kimata, Hajime. "Selective Enhancement of Production of Ige, Igg4, and Th2-Cell Cytokine During the Rebound Phenomenon in Atopic Dermatitis and Prevention by Suplatast Tosilate." *Annals of Allergy, Asthma & Immunology* 82, no. 3 (1999): 293-95.

[35] Fukaya, Mototsugu, Kenji Sato, Mitsuko Sato, Hajime Kimata, Shigeki Fujisawa, Haruhiko Dozono, Jun Yoshizawa, and Satoko Minaguchi. "Topical Steroid Addiction in Atopic Dermatitis." *Drug, healthcare and patient safety* 6 (2014): 131.

[36] Kligman, Albert M, and Peter J Frosch. "Steroid Addiction." *International journal of dermatology* 18, no. 1 (1979): 23-31.

[37] Jorissen, M, and Claus Bachert. "Effect of Corticosteroids on Wound Healing after Endoscopic Sinus Surgery." *Rhinology* 47, no. 3 (2009): 280.

[38] Hashimoto, Ichiro, Hideki Nakanishi, Yoshitaka Shono, Maki Toda, Hidetaka Tsuda, and Seiji Arase. "Angiostatic Effects of

Corticosteroid on Wound Healing of the Rabbit Ear." *Journal of Medical Investigation* 49, no. 1/2 (2002): 61-66.

[39] Martins, Manoela Domingues, Márcia Martins Marques, Sandra Kalil Bussadori, Marco Antonio Trevizani Martins, Vanessa Christina Santos Pavesi, Raquel Agnelli Mesquita-Ferrari, and Kristianne Porta Santos Fernandes. "Comparative Analysis between Chamomilla Recutita and Corticosteroids on Wound Healing. An in Vitro and in Vivo Study." *Phytotherapy Research: An International Journal Devoted to Pharmacological and Toxicological Evaluation of Natural Product Derivatives* 23, no. 2 (2009): 274-78.

[40] Abraham, Anil, and Gillian Roga. "Topical Steroid-Damaged Skin." *Indian journal of dermatology* 59, no. 5 (2014): 456.

[41] Gupta, Ratika, and Luz S. Fonacier. "Adverse Effects of Nonsystemic Steroids (Inhaled, Intranasal, and Cutaneous): A Review of the Literature and Suggested Monitoring Tool." *Current Allergy and Asthma Reports* 16, no. 6 (2016): 44.

[42] Kim, Hyun Jung, Hyun Jung Park, Jae Nam Yun, Se Kyoo Jeong, Sung Ku Ahn, and Seung Hun Lee. "Pseudoceramide-Containing Physiological Lipid Mixture Reduces Adverse Effects of Topical Steroids." *Allergy, asthma & immunology research* 3, no. 2 (2011): 96-102.

[43] Fisher, Louis B, and Howard I Maibach. "The Effect of Corticosteroids on Human Epidermal Mitotic Activity." *Archives of dermatology* 103, no. 1 (1971): 39-44.

[44] Marshall, Robert C, Michael Burrows, Leonard G Brookes, and Anthony Du Vivier. "The Effects of Topical and Systemic Glucocorticosteroids on DNA Synthesis in Different Tissues of the Hairless Mouse." *British Journal of Dermatology* 105, no. 5 (1981): 517-20.

[45] Sheu, Hamm-Ming, J Yu-Yun Lee, Kou-Wha Kuo, and Jui-Chen Tsai. "Permeability Barrier Abnormality of Hairless Mouse Epidermis after Topical Corticosteroid: Characterization of Stratum Corneum Lipids by Ruthenium Tetroxide Staining and High-

Performance Thin-Layer Chromatography." *The Journal of dermatology* 25, no. 5 (1998): 281-89.

[46] Stern, RS. "The Pattern of Topical Corticosteroid Prescribing in the United States, 1989-1991." *J Am Acad Dermatol* 35, no. 2 Pt 1 (1996): 183-6.

INDEX

A

B

C

D

E

F

G

H

I

J

K

L

M

N

O

P

Q

R

S

T

U

V

W

Z